T0322325

RECLAIMING YOU

RECLAIMING YOU

ABBY RAWLINSON

HAPPY BOOKS PLACE

Published in 2023 by Ebury Press, an imprint of Ebury Publishing
20 Vauxhall Bridge Road
London SW1V 2SA

Ebury Press is part of the Penguin Random House group of companies
whose addresses can be found at global.penguinrandomhouse.com

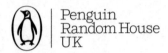

Penguin
Random House
UK

First published by Ebury Press in 2023

www.penguin.co.uk

A CIP catalogue record for this book is available from the British Library

ISBN 9781529908688
Typeset in Adobe Caslon Pro
Typeset by seagulls.net

Printed and bound in Great Britain by Clays Ltd, Elcograf S.p.A.

The authorised representative in the EEA is Penguin Random House
Ireland, Morrison Chambers, 32 Nassau Street, Dublin D02 YH68.

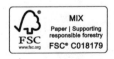

Penguin Random House is committed to a sustainable future
for our business, our readers and our planet. This book is made
from Forest Stewardship Council® certified paper.

For Andy and Beau

CONTENTS

INTRODUCTION: STARTING OUR JOURNEY

I will start by being totally honest with you. My job as a therapist isn't to 'fix' the people who walk through my door. They are not broken – and neither are you. My job is to help them find themselves – to come home to the person they've always been deep down, so that they can reclaim their confidence, their happiness and, ultimately, their life. My hope is that this book will help you do the same. As a therapist, I have never had someone arrive for their first therapy session and say, 'I'm here to reclaim my true self!' This is because most people don't realise how disconnected they have become from who they are at their core. More often than not, it is this disconnection between who they truly are and the person they are behaving as in daily life that is the key to resolving their problems. When my clients first come to see me, their disconnection from themselves is often disguised – it could be showing up as anxiety, feelings of imposter syndrome, trouble with boundaries, issues with motivation, people-pleasing or chronic busyness. But typically these are just signs that they have drifted from their true self.

I should probably tell you now that the words in this book are not going to tell you how to become a 'new you'. You've probably already read a few of those (I know I have!). Instead, I'm going to guide you through the process of gently stripping back your layers of self-protection to reveal the confident core that has been there all along. My hope is that the tools you find on these pages will help you to release some of the patterns that have been keeping you stuck, and to journey back to who you really are so you can live a more authentic, fulfilling and joyful life.

So many of us are disconnected from our true, authentic selves. Stress, trauma and the nature of our 'always on' modern lifestyles can push our minds and our bodies to their limits. Most of us believe that if we just try harder, think more positively or remove any negativity from our lives, that we'll be able to become unstuck, worry less, be happier, more balanced and have healthier relationships. Yet, our anxiety, exhaustion, loneliness and resentment persist. Why are we so stuck? I believe that, in a large part, it's because we can't just *think* our way towards feeling better and more connected: we need to look at the mind and body as a whole.

When we neglect our needs and ignore what our bodies are telling us, we're unintentionally keeping our nervous systems in 'survival mode', a state in which we can feel anxious and on-edge or withdrawn and exhausted. This state is one of our body's most powerful protective mechanisms, designed to help us cope with extreme, occasional situations. But the more time we spend living in a dysregulated state, with our nervous system out of balance, the more disconnected we become from our true self. We have made it 'normal' to exist in survival mode and it means we're preventing ourselves from being the fullest, happiest expression of ourselves.

I am an integrative therapist, which means I'm trained in more than one therapeutic modality. When I work with my clients, I integrate the different tools, strategies and principles of various therapeutic approaches, from cognitive behavioural therapy (CBT) and psychodynamic psychotherapy to mindfulness and somatic, or body-based therapy. Essentially, I don't believe that one theory has the magic answer. Above all, I view my clients as a whole being, not just a brain. The word 'integrative' comes from the Latin word *integer*, which means to make whole, to complete.

Throughout this book, you will learn how to bring a mind–body perspective to overcoming life's twists and turns, and blend elements from many different practices to help you uncover your true self. In my experience, the most profound life changes occur when we harness the power of the psychological, the emotional *and* the physical. This integrative, holistic approach reflects the recent paradigm shift in how we view and treat mental health. Many great thinkers have opened our eyes to the new science of the mind-body connection and the role it plays in how we feel, act and think.

HARNESSING THE POWER OF THE PSYCHOLOGICAL, THE EMOTIONAL AND THE PHYSICAL CAN LEAD TO THE MOST PROFOUND LIFE CHANGES.

OUR MIND AND BODY

When I say it's important to think about our bodies, this doesn't mean I'm going to tell you that getting more sleep, exercising and eating more vegetables is going to make you feel better; you already know this. Instead, I'm going to begin by introducing you to your nervous system and showing you how to repair and regulate it, so that you can develop more resilience, and more control over how you feel. In my experience, this is the deepest mind–body healing work we can do – it is the foundation to reclaiming your whole, authentic self.

Why is our nervous system central to reclaiming our true selves? When our nervous system is regulated and balanced, we flow with life's ups and downs – we are resilient. We are comfortable to be our most true selves because we feel *safe*. In contrast, when our nervous system is dysregulated and we are living in survival mode, we respond to everyday challenges as if they are life or death situations. We don't have the space to hear our authentic selves.

I remember when I first learned the importance of our nervous systems in my training to be a therapist. It was in a module on body psychotherapy and initially, I was a bit sceptical. At the beginning of each class, the lecturer would go around the room and each student had to describe any sensations they had noticed in their body throughout the week. Some of my peers would say they had noticed tightness in their jaw when they had conflict with their partner, or a buzzy feeling in their chest when they felt stressed at work, and they would be able to attach these sensations to what state their nervous system was in. But me, I couldn't do it. I felt nothing. I was disconnected from my body sensations because I lived purely in my head. I had no problem articulating my thoughts, but describing what was going on in my body felt impossible.

A SENSE OF SAFETY IS INTEGRAL TO THE JOURNEY OF SELF-DISCOVERY.

Weirdly, I initially viewed this disconnection from my body as a strength: I could push through stressful experiences without getting distracted by sensations in my body and I could still be highly productive when I was tired or anxious. But throughout the training, as my body awareness grew, I realised that being able to listen to cues from my body was a superpower: I became more in control of my thoughts and feelings, I could handle stress more smoothly and I was able to consistently show up for myself and my own needs. It felt like a revelation, and by the end of this book you'll have all the tools you need to do the same.

WHERE WE GO WRONG – OUR BARRIERS TO AUTHENTICITY

Once you start to turn inwards and connect with the innate wisdom your body has to offer, you may come to realise that you've been spending a lot of your time living in survival mode. You may even start to notice that some of the behaviours you thought were helping you have actually kept you feeling stuck and stressed out.

For example, many of us falsely believe that if we can keep everyone around us happy, ignore our painful feelings, stay small, stay busy, or strive for perfection then we'll feel safe, loved and happy. These coping strategies act like a protective shell around our true self. But it's a self-defeating protective shell. Rather than protecting us, these coping strategies further dysregulate our nervous systems, and further disconnect us from ourselves and the people around us.

These coping strategies take many different forms. Maybe you find yourself saying yes to an extra project at work and taking on more than you can comfortably manage because you don't want to let people down. Or maybe you find yourself running your decisions past everyone because you're worried about making the 'wrong' choice or being criticised. Or maybe you find yourself saying, 'It's fine,' when a comment has hurt your feelings, because you want to keep the peace and avoid being disliked. We've all experienced moments like these – but it's when these inauthentic expressions become habitual patterns of behaviour that we can really lose track of ourselves and wind up feeling disconnected, burnt out and resentful. Within the pages of this book, we're going to look at why we develop these unhelpful coping strategies, but, more than that, we are going to look at what we can do about it.

WHAT YOU WILL FIND IN THIS BOOK

Reclaiming You is structured in three parts. The first part provides the foundations for reconnecting with your true self – getting to know your nervous system. This part of the book will offer practical and actionable steps to help you tune in and regulate your nervous system. I'll guide you through the process of identifying your 'triggers' (what prompts dysregulated states) and 'glimmers' (the actions that help you soothe your nervous system) so that you can start to develop more resilience and control over how you feel in your day-to-day life. This is the foundation to living a full, happy and authentic life.

Part 2 is all about the barriers to being your true self – the roadblocks to your authenticity. Because we can't fully reclaim our true self until we understand the things that get in the way. We'll break down the most common unhealthy coping strategies we employ to cope with the pressures of life – from people-pleasing and perfectionism to numbing and chronic busyness – and look at the ways to address them, so that you can dismantle your protective shell, piece by piece. When you can let go of the coping behaviours and habits that are keeping you hidden, stressed and resentful, you can gain access to your true self – the 'you' that feels enough, just as you are.

In Part 3, we will learn to apply all the knowledge you've gained in order to fully reclaim your true self. I'll teach you the long-term skills and strategies you need to shrink your inner critic, find your voice, consistently take care of yourself, and set your boundaries without feeling guilty, so that you can finally reclaim your time, your confidence, and your life. I believe it's absolutely possible to live life feeling more connected and in tune with our authentic selves. And I tell you, once you start to reconnect with your internal world, you'll be amazed at how things start to change in your external world too.

Let's get started.

PART 1

GETTING TO KNOW YOUR NERVOUS SYSTEM

1.
A REAL-WORLD UNDERSTANDING OF THE NERVOUS SYSTEM

Have you ever felt your heart race if you've had to swerve to avoid a collision on the motorway? Or felt your palms sweat when there is turbulence on a flight? Or have you ever felt your body freeze in fear when, for a split second, that pile of clothes on your bedroom chair looks like a murderer?

If you answered yes to any of these questions, then you have experienced your nervous system in action. You see, the human body is pretty well designed – it wants you to have a healthy fear of things that could be dangerous.

When you think of your autonomic nervous system, you may have a distant memory of GCSE biology lessons and recall that this system has something to do with 'fight or flight'. And you would be correct. This is connected to the autonomic nervous system's primary function: to ensure we survive in moments of danger. It's a system that acts largely outside of our conscious awareness and is responsible for regulating our bodily functions such as circulation, respiration and digestion. I like to think of the autonomic nervous system as the body's main operating system: It's critical to our survival; it runs 24 hours a day; and it's doing its thing even when we're not paying attention in the slightest.

To get a better understanding of how your nervous system works to keep you safe, let's imagine you are living in the hunter-gatherer days. Suppose something life-threatening happens, like, say, being chased by a lion. Your nervous system would automatically switch on the fight-or-flight response and your body would immediately prepare to engage in an attack (fight), or alternatively, running away (flight). To allow for this, your heart would beat faster, your breath would become shallower and your digestion would slow down. Adrenaline, cortisol and norepinephrine – known as the three stress hormones – would be released into your bloodstream, and everything in your body and mind would become focused on the impending danger. Then, after the danger of the lion had passed, the switch would go off and your nervous system would return to a calm and relaxed state.

The problem is, we're not living the hunter-gatherer life any more. Most of us have never been chased by a lion, but our body thinks it's happening all the time. Even as you read this now, it's possible that your body is in fight-or-flight mode. Your nervous system may be mistaking daily stressors – like an inbox full of emails, or a delayed train – for a lion. That is because whether the threat is a low-grade mini-drama or a life-or-death situation, the body just does its job of trying to keep you safe. Essentially, fight-or-flight mode can be triggered unnecessarily – in the same way as an oversensitive burglar alarm.

This stress response is a beautiful system, designed to keep us safe – but we are not meant to stay in fight-or-flight mode for extended periods of time. If our nervous system stays in survival mode for too long, or if we're constantly in and out of it, it can play havoc with our physical and emotional well-being. We need to process our stress or discharge it; otherwise it just builds up and builds up, and we start to experience the consequences, often in the form of anxiety, chronic stress and burnout.

The three states of the nervous system

So far, for the sake of simplicity, I have talked about the nervous system as having two states: these are called the sympathetic system, or fight-or-flight (activated when the lion appears) and the parasympathetic system, or returning to relaxation (activated when the threat of the lion has passed). The two sides of the system are equal and opposite, complementing each other like yin and yang. Your parasympathetic is your 'rest and digest' state, where you feel calm and at peace, your body can heal, rebuild, give birth here: this is where we are when we feel safe. The sympathetic state is the fight-or-flight state, where we are facing a threat and poised for action; where we feel in danger. However, recent research has changed our understanding of how the nervous system works beyond these two states. In 1994, psychologist Stephen Porges brought forth a new and illuminating model of the nervous system, known as Polyvagal Theory.

Thanks to Porges' work, we now know that there are actually *three* states of the autonomic nervous system, which not only regulate the workings of our body but also our emotional states. Alongside the sympathetic nervous system, polyvagal theory

The 3 States of the Nervous System

① **Safe-and-social**

This is the relaxed state we are in when we feel safe, calm and happy

② **Fight-or-flight**

This is the state we are in when we feel anxious, stressed or angry

③ **Shutdown**

This is the state we are in when we feel low, detached or unmotivated outlines that the parasympathetic nervous system is split into two distinct branches: a '**ventral vagal system**', or safe-and-social, which supports social engagement, and a '**dorsal vagal system**', or 'shutdown', which encourages defensive immobilisation.

Everyone experiences all three nervous system states, and we can move in and out of each state every single day, sometimes multiple times a day. Becoming aware of which nervous system state we are in at any given moment is incredibly useful for our mental health because each state has a different impact on how we think and feel.

When I first learned about the three different states of the nervous system from reading Deb Dana's book *Polyvagal Theory in Therapy*, I had a big 'ah-ha' moment. I suddenly understood my shifting moods and thinking patterns in a new and profound way. I agree with Deb Dana that there is a 'before and after' element to learning this theory. Once you know how the nervous system shapes our lives, you can never again *not* see your experience through this lens.

The nervous system as a whole is a continuum – we can experience the different states of the system in both small and big ways. A small visit to fight-or-flight might feel like slight edginess or alertness, whereas a more intense visit might be a full-blown panic attack. Similarly with shutdown: at the lower end of the spectrum you may feel a bit flat and unmotivated, but in a more extreme case you might experience dissociation (where you feel detached from your body and the world). We can also experience different degrees of safe-and-social, ranging from feeling a general sense of ease, to feeling full-blown bliss. On our journey to reclaiming ourselves, it's crucial we have an understanding of all three states and the varying degrees to which they can show up in our lives. Here's what you need to know:

1. The safe-and-social state – ventral vagal system

This is the state we're in when we feel happy, relaxed and grounded. When we're in the safe-and-social state, our nervous system is regulated: we feel positive and life feels manageable. Instead of freaking out over life's small inconveniences, we are able to 'go with the flow' and see the bigger picture. So when we miss the bus or our phone battery dies, we can still meet the demands of the day without getting overwhelmed.

When our nervous system is in this regulated state, we can be compassionate towards ourselves and to others, we can experience feelings of love and friendship, and we're comfortable with both being alone or with other people. The safe-and-social state is the 'sweet spot' and our preferred place to be. It's the place where we can be our most true and authentic selves.

---

10 SIGNS YOU ARE IN THE VENTRAL, SAFE-AND-SOCIAL STATE:

- You feel safe, calm and present

- You have a general sense of 'everything is OK'

- You can be productive and creative

- You feel comfortable and secure being in your own company or being with others

- You feel clear-headed and able to focus

- You feel capable of handling whatever comes your way

- You trust yourself and the world around you

- You are able to collaborate with others

- Your thoughts tend to be compassionate and curious, rather than critical and rigid

- You can be organised and follow through with plans

2. Fight-or-flight – sympathetic system

When our mind and body perceive a threat, we move into the fight-or-flight state. The threat that moves us here might be a real danger, like seeing a big truck barrelling towards us as we cross the road, or a perceived threat, like an influx of messages pinging at us through email and WhatsApp. From an evolutionary perspective, we enter fight-or-flight mode when our system thinks the best course of action is to fight or run away but we tend to experience it as anger or anxiety.

Being in fight-or-flight mode can be a fleeting experience, but many of us are *living* in this activated state. When fight-or-flight mode is an everyday norm for us, it can feel like we are existing in a constant state of emergency. We lose our sense of feeling safe and everything seems dangerous or urgent. We jump out of our skin when the doorbell rings or we find it impossible to slow down and stop working, even if we are exhausted.

This is also the mode we are in when we impulsively react to people rather than thoughtfully respond to them. This might look like snapping at our loved ones or firing off passive-aggressive emails to our colleagues without pausing to reflect on the potential impact. When we are in fight-or-flight mode, we can usually feel it in our body – we might feel shaky or dizzy, experience heart palpitations, tightness in the chest or feel out of breath.

SIGNS YOU ARE IN THE SYMPATHETIC FIGHT-OR-FLIGHT STATE:

- You feel anxious, stressed, frustrated or angry
- You feel out of sync with others
- You are consumed by racing/worried thoughts, and you struggle to sleep
- You feel on-edge and 'jumpy'
- The world feels like a dangerous place
- Your energy feels chaotic
- You feel irritable or snappy
- You find it difficult to focus or sit still
- It feels impossible to 'go with the flow'
- You feel like everyone is being unfriendly
- Everything seems urgent and it feels impossible to 'slow down'
- You feel tired but unable to switch off and relax

3. Shutdown – dorsal vagal system

If we continue to feel trapped in a cycle of stress, with no way to manage, we go into the shutdown state. Here, life's never-ending challenges no longer seem to matter and we begin to withdraw and disconnect from ourselves and others around us. This is the state we're in when we feel depressed, hopeless, and have no energy to do even the simplest of things.

As with all states of the nervous system, the time spent here can be fleeting. But when we are living in shutdown mode it can be a struggle to get out of bed or feel motivated. It's like we have no energy to care. We might forget to reply to an important text or we might zone-out when someone is talking to us. In shutdown mode, we can feel so heavy and stuck that even reaching for a glass of water when we're thirsty, or plugging in our phone when the battery is dying, can feel like almost impossible tasks. When we are in this state of collapse, we feel numb, foggy or heavy, and instead of wanting to connect with people, we want to hide away and not move.

SIGNS YOU ARE IN THE DORSAL
SHUTDOWN STATE:

- You feel depressed, withdrawn, foggy or numb

- You feel spaced-out

- You feel hopeless and self-critical

- You have little energy or motivation

- You feel disconnected from yourself, others, and the world

- You have no energy or desire to connect with people

- You are on 'autopilot' mode, where you feel like you're just moving through life with little awareness

- You want to hide away from the world

- You feel like a misfit, or like you don't belong

- You struggle to set goals or do anything creative

- You have difficulty remembering details or making decisions

- You feel invisible or like you've disappeared

- You feel 'not here' and unreachable

The shutdown state is also sometimes referred to as 'freeze'. This is because it's the system that's activated when our mind and body decide that the best course of action is to be quiet and still. Just like the fight-or-flight response, the shutdown response is an automatic, involuntary response to a threat. It's our body deciding in a split-second that immobilisation, or freezing – rather than fighting or running away – is the best way to survive what's happening. We see this in animals who suddenly stop moving and 'play dead' as a last-ditch attempt at survival (which can work because predators will typically lose interest in an animal that is already dead).

In humans, there can be a lot of shame and confusion associated with the shutdown response. Even though it's a common response, it's not as well-known as fight-or-flight. Many people who have experienced the more extreme end of the shutdown spectrum will look back at a situation where they were unsafe or scared and wonder why they didn't shout, kick or run away. The truth is they *couldn't* fight or run. Going into shutdown mode is not a cognitive decision; it's an automatic physiological response. There is nothing 'wrong' with you for freezing – your body made its best effort to keep you alive.

However, remaining chronically in shutdown mode, at any end of the spectrum, when there is no longer any threat can be detrimental to our health and well-being. It robs us of our joy, productivity and ability to connect with others. When you come out of a shutdown state, you may feel ashamed and guilty, but it's important to remember that 'shutdown' doesn't mean you're lazy or incompetent; it means you're stuck in a dysregulated state.

How our minds react - the flavour of our thoughts

As you'll have seen from the lists above, our emotions and body sensations can give us a lot of information about the state of our nervous system. In the next chapter, we'll look at how we can physically soothe our bodies and our nervous systems. But first, let's take a look at how to identify our thinking patterns when we're in each state, and what we can do to stop unhelpful thinking in fight-or-flight and shutdown states. I find it really helpful to break this down by identifying the flavour of our thoughts, noticing if we're thinking: 'I can', 'I must' or 'I can't'.

When we are in the safe-and-social state, and life feels manageable, our thoughts typically have an 'I can' flavour to them. For example, our thoughts might be along the lines of *'I can do this'* or *'everything is going to be OK'*. When we are in this nervous system 'sweet zone', we have a mindset of possibility and choice.

However, when something threatens our sense of safety – whether it is real or imagined – and we move into the fight-or-flight state, our thoughts tend to feel urgent and have an 'I must' flavour to them. We might have thoughts like '*I must work harder*' or '*I need to get out of here right now*'. Our mindset is 'go, go, go', with a focus on action.

When our system decides that the best strategy to survive a threat is to stop and disconnect, we move into the shutdown state. This is where we can feel flat or numb, and our internal dialogue can be about being alone, unseen or unwanted. Our thoughts here can feel slow and tend to have an 'I can't' flavour to them. We might have thoughts like '*I'm useless, I just want to disappear*', or '*there's no point in even trying*'.

Once you start recognising the flavour of your thoughts, you will probably notice that the thoughts you have in the dysregulated fight-or-flight and shutdown states tend to be dramatic and absolute. These are called 'cognitive distortions' in psychology – it's a term that means the way you are thinking about something doesn't necessarily match up to the reality of what is going on. We all have some cognitive distortions, but they are particularly common, and tricky to shift, when our nervous system is dysregulated. When you suspect you might be in either fight-or-flight or shutdown mode, it can be useful to see if any of these distortions resonate with you.

5 Types of Cognitive Distortion

Black and white thinking

Jumping to conclusions

Catastrophising

Personalising

Negative focus

FIVE TYPES OF COGNITIVE DISTORTIONS THAT TEND TO ARISE WHEN OUR NERVOUS SYSTEM IS DYSREGULATED:

- **Black and white thinking:** You see things in absolutes and there is no middle ground - you ignore the 'shades of grey'. Either you do things perfectly or it's a complete waste of time. This can lead to 'Always or Never' thinking where you assume that from one bad experience that all similar situations will always be the same. For example: *'Nobody at work likes me'* or *'I always say the wrong thing'*.

- **Jumping to conclusions:** This is when you jump to conclusions without finding out all of the facts. This can lead you to start predicting the future or becoming a mind-reader where you assume that you know other people's thoughts, intentions and motives. For example: *'She thinks I'm useless at my job'*; or *'I'm going to get fired'*.

- **Personalising:** This is when you take responsibility and blame for anything unpleasant, even if it has nothing to do with you. Events or situations are interpreted as indicators of something negative about you, when in fact they may have nothing to do with you. For example: *'It's my fault the meeting went badly'*; or *'I'm the reason he's miserable'*.

- **Catastrophising:** This is when you magnify and exaggerate the importance of events and how awful they could be. This leads to over-estimating the chances of disaster, ending with thoughts like *'whatever will go wrong will go wrong'*.

For example: *'I'm going to mess this up and get fired'*; or *'We're going to break-up and I'm going to have nowhere to live'*.

- **Negative Focus:** This is where you focus on the negative, ignoring or misinterpreting positive aspects of the situation. If you have done a good job, you filter this out and reject the positive comments and focus on your negative thoughts. For example: *'My annual review was completely terrible'*; or *'I didn't say anything right in that meeting'*.

HOW TO STOP NEGATIVE THOUGHT SPIRALS

Cognitive distortions are often at the beginning of a negative 'thought spiral', a term to describe when an initial negative thought has us sinking further and further into a dysregulated state of fight-or-flight or shutdown. The more we listen to these irrational thoughts, the more dysregulated our nervous system can become. Our thinking informs our physical reactions and vice versa.

While it may not always feel like it, we do have control over how much power a thought has. We can decide how much we are going to buy into it. Thoughts are not facts! They are predictions, stories, memories or theories. Sometimes just having the awareness of the cognitive distortion will be enough to remind us that our thought is fake news. But other irrational thoughts are more habitual or deeply ingrained and will require a little extra work in the form of 'thought-correcting'. This is the process of challenging your thoughts by asking yourself five 'magic questions':

If You're Having Negative Thoughts, Ask Yourself...

'What is the evidence that this thought is true?'

'Am I viewing this situation as black and white, when really it's more complicated?'

'Am I having this thought because I'm in fight-or-flight/shutdown, or do facts support it?'

'If the worst did happen, what could I do to cope with it or handle it?'

'What would I tell a friend if they had the same thought?'

Once we start challenging our thoughts with the magic questions, we can start to reframe our thoughts into something more realistic and nuanced, and tell ourselves a more helpful, compassionate story.

Thought-correcting is about looking for words that shift our thoughts and stories in the direction of autonomic safety, where we feel regulated and clear-headed. In fight-or-flight or shutdown, our thoughts have a narrow focus, but when we're in a safe-and-social state of regulation, we have a more nuanced view of things.

The words we choose can have a powerful impact on the state of our nervous system, but thought-correcting is a skill that takes practice so don't be too hard on yourself if you don't get it right away. Our brains have become addicted to only noticing what is wrong and what is dangerous. And, as with most addictions, breaking this deeply entrenched habit can take time.

NEXT TIME YOU FEEL YOURSELF REPEATING A NEGATIVE THOUGHT TO YOURSELF AS IF IT'S A FACT, HAVE A GO AT REFRAMING IT BY GOING THROUGH THE FIVE MAGIC QUESTIONS.

I'm not exaggerating when I say that I have thought-corrected thousands of my own negative thoughts. The day I received the news that I would be able to write this book, I also found out that I was pregnant with my first child. Straight away I was thinking '*This is too much*' and I started started catastrophising: What if I have a difficult pregnancy and I'm too sick to write

Reframing 'Fight-Or-Flight' Thoughts

THOUGHT

REFRAME AFTER ASKING THE MAGIC QUESTIONS

'I must never mess up or I'll be harshly judged and criticised' ⟹ 'Mistakes are part of being human. Nothing is ever perfect'

'My boss hasn't replied. She must be mad at me' ⟹ 'There could be multiple reasons why my boss hasn't replied. Jumping to conclusions and catastrophising is making me anxious'

'I can't trust anyone to help me' 'Not allowing other people to support me can lead to stress and burnout'

Reframing 'Shutdown' Thoughts

THOUGHT	REFRAME AFTER ASKING THE MAGIC QUESTIONS
'Everyone thinks I'm useless at my job'	'Just because I feel I'm not good enough, it doesn't mean I'm right'
'I don't belong here'	'Everyone shares the same fears and insecurities. I deserve to be here'
'I'm so lazy'	'This situation has been difficult for me and I have needed to rest'

the book? What if I find writing too stressful and I make myself ill and burnt out? I had to immediately reframe these thoughts into something more realistic to prevent a downward sprial into panic. Confronting our negative thoughts quickly is essential in reconnecting with our true selves because a single unchallenged negative thought can rage out of control and become toxic if it isn't confronted and corrected.

EXERCISE: GETTING FAMILIAR WITH HOW YOU THINK AND FEEL

This is an exercise to help you gently get to know your nervous system and your thinking patterns. In a notebook or on a device, write down your answers to these three questions:

1. *What is it like when I am in my regulated safe-and-social state (ventral vagal)?*

2. *What is it like when I'm in my dysregulated fight-or-flight state (sympathetic)?*

3. *What is it like when I am in my dysregulated shutdown state (dorsal vagal)?*

For all three questions, include notes on your sensations, thoughts and feelings.

For example:

When I'm in my safe-and-social state, I feel alive, open and spacious in my body. I feel clear-headed, happy and relaxed, and my thoughts tend to be along the lines of, 'I can do this', 'I have everything I need'.

When I'm in my fight-or-flight state, I feel tightness in my chest, tension in my shoulders and heat in my neck. I feel anxious, irritable and panicky, and my thoughts tend to be along the lines of 'I'm so overwhelmed', 'I can't make any mistakes'.

When I'm in my shutdown state, I feel foggy, cold, and heavy in my body. I feel disconnected, numb and low, and my thoughts tend to be along the lines of 'I'm lazy and useless', 'What's the point in trying?'

This exercise can be challenging, so remember to be kind and patient with yourself! You might find tuning into your body and naming the sensations particularly difficult and uncomfortable but try not to skip this part.

The ability to pay attention to body-based sensations is called 'interoception', and it's a fundamental part of getting to know your nervous system and recognising which state you're in. If you're struggling to find the language, here is a list of common sensory words you might want to choose from:

Achy	Closed	Empty
Airy	Constricted	Energised
Alive	Contracted	Expansive
Blocked	Cold	Fluid
Breathless	Dense	Frozen
Bubbly	Dizzy	Foggy
Buzzing	Dull	Full

Flushed	Paralysed	Stretched
Fluttery	Pressure	Strong
Hard	Prickly	Sweaty
Hot	Pulsing	Thick
Heavy Intense	Quiet	Tightness
Jittery	Quivery	Tense
Jumpy	Radiating	Tight
Knotted	Shaky	Tingly
Light	Shivery	Trembly
Loose	Sharp	Warm
Limp	Smooth	Wobbly
Numb	Soft	Weak
Open	Spacious	

2.
THREATS TO OUR NERVOUS SYSTEM: TRIGGERS

You may not realise it, but as you walk around in the world each day, your nervous system is constantly scanning your environment for cues of safety or danger: *should I be careful here? Is this person safe? Is this a threatening situation?* To do this, your nervous system uses something called 'neuroception': a 'sixth sense' that acts below your level of conscious awareness. It's an ongoing process and a true gift, designed to keep us alive.

As we covered in the previous chapter, when your autonomic nervous system perceives a situation as safe, you enter the safe-and-social state, where you feel peaceful, happy, and able to connect with others. However, when you feel a sense of unease, or you perceive a threat to your well-being, your body activates the survival modes of fight-or-flight or shutdown. From a nervous system perspective, these threats are called 'triggers'.

A trigger can be a real threat (like seeing a car suddenly pull out in front of you) or a perceived threat (like receiving a blunt email from your boss). Triggers are why we can suddenly go from feeling 'OK' to 'not OK'.

TRIGGERS ARE THE PEOPLE, PLACES, THINGS OR SITUATIONS THAT CREATE A SENSE OF DANGER AND ACTIVATE THE NERVOUS SYSTEM'S DEFENCES.

So, if triggers are the things that move us into fight-or-flight and shutdown responses, what are the things that can move us into a regulated safe-and-social state? These things are known as 'glimmers', which is a beautiful term coined by therapist and nervous system specialist, Deb Dana.

Glimmers are the opposite of triggers. They are the experiences, interactions, or resources that help us feel safe and settled. They are moments of safety that help calm the nervous system and return us to a regulated state. Glimmers can be interactions with others, like a phone call with a friend or a hug from a loved one, or they can be solo experiences, like walking in nature or watching your favourite TV show.

Glimmers activate a part of the body called the vagus nerve; this is known as the 'care-taking', or wandering nerve, Vagus is the Latin word for wandering. The vagus nerve begins in the core of the brain and wanders all the way into the gut – it is responsible for getting us back into a state, where we feel calm, focused and at ease. Remember how we discussed Polyvagal Theory, on page 13. Polyvagal Theory is based around the understanding of the role of the vagus nerve in emotion regulation, social connection and fear response.

A REAL-WORLD EXAMPLE OF TRIGGERS AND GLIMMERS

To give you a better sense of how triggers and glimmers work, here is a real-world description of how someone might move in and out of the different nervous system states throughout the day. I've taken inspiration here from Deb Dana's description of the Polyvagal Ladder.

Let's say I'm walking to work in the morning. The sun is shining, I'm listening to some amazing music, and I'm feeling good – my nervous system is in the safe-and-social state. Then I trip. I spill coffee down my top and the contents of my bag pours out onto the pavement. This mini-drama startles my nervous system and triggers the fight-or-flight response. My heart rate increases, my breath becomes shallow and all I can focus on is gathering up my belongings and leaving the scene without drawing any more attention to myself. I start walking again and I feel embarrassed, shaky and consumed by worried thoughts about my coffee-stained top.

When I get to work, I remember I have a spare top so I get changed and I feel a wave of relief. I sit down at my desk and say hello to my colleagues. My heart rate starts to settle and I no longer feel like a flustered, sweaty mess. I tell my colleagues about my journey to work and they say a few sympathetic and kind words that put me at ease. I feel seen and understood and my nervous system feels calm again. I notice that I feel clear-headed and able to focus – I'm back in the safe-and-social state. My nervous system is regulated again.

In a meeting later that day, my boss makes a comment that irritates me. The more I listen to him talk, the angrier I feel. I notice my heart rate increasing and my cheeks becoming hot. I feel like I want to either shout at him or storm out of the room – I'm back in my dysregulated fight-or-flight state. Someone asks me a question and as soon as I start to respond, my boss interrupts and talks over me. I stay quiet and as the meeting carries on around me, I disconnect from the conversation. I feel ignored, invisible and undervalued. I feel like there is no point in me being there. Now I'm going into shutdown mode.

The meeting ends and I go back to my desk. I stay quiet for the rest of the afternoon. I feel unmotivated and low in energy, with no desire to talk to anyone. I just want to go home and hide from the world. I feel stuck in the collapsed state of shutdown.

When I get home, I have a bath and listen to my favourite podcast. I start to feel a bit more alive and energised. I notice that I'm taking deeper breaths and my thoughts are a bit more positive. I'm heading towards the safe-and-social state. When I get out of the bath, I call my friend and tell her about what happened today with my boss. She empathises with me and I feel heard and understood. She shares some of the frustrations she has with her own boss and I notice I feel compassion towards her. When I hang up, I take a deep sigh and I feel a sense of 'everything is OK' wash over me. I no longer feel alone – I'm fully back in a regulation.

In this story, there are a few different triggers that create a sense of danger and activate my nervous system's defences. Tripping and spilling my coffee was the first trigger, which dysregulated my system towards fight-or-flight. Then later, the annoying comment from my boss was a trigger, pulling me, once again, into fight-or-flight. The final trigger was my boss making me feel ignored, which sent me into shutdown mode.

There are also multiple glimmers in this story that helped regulate my system and moved me back into a calm and connected state. Talking to my colleagues when I arrived at work put me at ease and sent me straight back into safe-and-social mode. Then later, when I was in the shutdown state, it was the bath and listening to my favourite podcast that created an upward spiral of regulation. Then finally, the kind words from my friend acted as a glimmer and moved me fully into regulation, where the world felt safe again.

HOW TO IDENTIFY YOUR TRIGGERS

It's important to know that identifying your triggers and glimmers won't stop you from experiencing the fight-or-flight and shutdown responses. These systems are beautifully designed to protect us and keep us safe. But being in tune with what pulls us into a survival response and what sends us towards safety can help us feel more in control when difficult moments inevitably do happen. When we understand that some of our behaviour is a result of automatic responses rather than cognitive choices, we can soften an inner critic that shames and blames us, and invite more self-compassion into our lives.

Becoming attuned to ourselves and recognising which state our nervous system is in is key to helping us reconnect with our true selves. The sense of predictability that comes with knowing what our triggers and our glimmers are can help us make sense of our thoughts, feelings and behaviours. It empowers us to harness our nervous system to work for us rather than against us.

Not only is this a game-changer for our mental health and our relationships, but it is an essential step to becoming our most comfortable and whole selves. When we understand how our nervous system works, we can change our mindset from '*this is how I am*' to '*this is how I respond*'. It's a subtle difference but it's a huge step towards becoming more self-aware and reclaiming our confidence.

For some people, moving out of fight-or-flight or shut-down can be difficult, and they can get stuck in dysregulated states. This is when we need to work towards healing the nervous system, which we'll look at in the next chapter.

Physical triggers

Once you start paying attention to your nervous system, you will start to recognise your triggers, and you will begin to understand why your survival response is being activated in certain situations. Your triggers might be *real* threats, when your life is in actual danger (like hearing a smoke alarm in the middle of the night) or *perceived* threats, when your body has a felt-sense of danger (like needing to have a difficult conversation with an employee).

Emotional Triggers

However, there may be situations where you feel triggered (in other words, dysregulated) and you can't understand why. You might enter survival mode when nothing scary or stressful is happening. For example, maybe your partner forgets to buy the kind of bread you like and out of nowhere you feel overwhelmed with anger. You might think to yourself, '*Why am I going into fight-or-flight mode right now? It's just bread; it's not a big deal.*' An overly dramatic reaction like this is normally the result of an emotional trigger.

AN EMOTIONAL TRIGGER IS ANYTHING
- INCLUDING PLACES, EXPERIENCES,
OR EVENTS - THAT UNCONSCIOUSLY
REMINDS US OF OLD PAINFUL FEELINGS
OR PAST TRAUMAS, TYPICALLY FROM
OUR CHILDHOOD.

Emotional triggers can be confusing because they spark an intense emotional reaction that can feel disproportionate to what is actually going on.

Let's look at the bread example. If you did a bit of exploration into your intense reaction to the wrong bread, you might discover it's not *actually* about the bread. It might be about a childhood pattern of being denied the things you enjoy. Or perhaps you are experiencing some unprocessed frustration about not feeling listened to by a parent.

Because an emotional trigger sends our body into fight-or-flight or shutdown, we can often lose touch with our healthy coping skills when we are triggered, particularly when we don't understand the trigger. It's times like these when we can succumb to reacting rather than reflecting and responding.

When we are triggered in this way, we are experiencing past pain in the present moment. It's like the reopening of a wound that hasn't had a chance to heal. Our emotional triggers tend to be based on our personal histories and although they are completely unique to us, there are some common triggers to look out for.

SOME COMMON EXAMPLES OF EMOTIONAL TRIGGERS:

- You might get angry when you think you are being told what to do if you felt controlled in the past

- You might get anxious whenever someone isn't there for you if you had emotionally unavailable parents

- You might feel intense sadness when you are excluded, if your parents often ignored your needs

- You might panic when you are in a situation over which you have no control if you have a history of feeling helpless

---

If we look at my earlier example of being interrupted by my boss in a meeting, it was the feeling of being ignored that triggered me and sent me into shutdown state, where I felt invisible and hopeless. For some people, feeling ignored might trigger the fight-or-flight response, where you feel angry or anxious. For others, it might not trigger a defence response at all. Everyone's emotional triggers are different because we have all had unique life experiences.

A useful saying to remember when it comes to emotional triggers is, 'If it's hysterical, it's historical', which I first heard from Karamo Brown on an episode of *Queer Eye*. Meaning, if you are blowing something out of proportion, it's most likely because of something in your past.

The wonderful thing about being able to recognise our triggers as they happen is that it can enable us to consciously choose coping skills and glimmers to regulate our system. When I felt triggered by my boss ignoring me, I went back to my desk, stayed quiet, and sank further into my shutdown response. If I had been able to recognise that I had been triggered, I could have asked myself if there was anything I could to do to regulate my system. I may have decided to go on a walk, call a friend, or done some deep breathing exercises – all of which could have lifted me out of my shutdown state and moved me into regulation. If I had been able to recognise that I was triggered and then participate in an activity that regulated my nervous system, I could have spent the rest of the afternoon in a safe-and-social state where I felt focused and productive.

When our nervous system returns to a regulated state after being triggered, we can sometimes feel ashamed, guilty or confused about how we felt or behaved. From a place of calm and safety, our reactions may seem irrational. It's important to remember that it's not a bad thing to have these extreme reactions – often it's an opportunity to do some more grieving or to heal some things from the past that have been simmering under the surface and need to be dealt with.

Why Was I Triggered?

I felt
ignored

I felt
blamed

I felt
trapped

I felt
manipulated

I felt
judged

I felt
unheard

I felt
controlled

I felt
unsupported

I felt
helpless

EXERCISE: HOW TO IDENTIFY YOUR EMOTIONAL TRIGGERS

Identifying our emotional triggers can be broken down into a simple four-step process:

1. Notice the internal shift

It's not always easy to recognise what has triggered us. Our heightened emotions and dysregulated nervous system can make it difficult to pinpoint what exactly stimulated such a strong response. To identify your trigger, go back and try to find the exact moment when you went from 'OK' to 'not OK'. What felt upsetting? Was it a comment from your dad? A story on the news? A text from a friend? Write this down.

2. Next, name your feelings, thoughts and sensations

Then, notice how you *felt* when you were triggered. Did you feel sad, anxious, scared, angry? What did you feel in your body? Hot, tense, heavy or slow? What were your thoughts like? Did they have an 'I must' or an 'I can't' flavour to them? If you're struggling for words to describe how you feel in your body, go back to page 32 where there's a list that can be helpful for putting your bodily sensations into words.

3. Then, name the autonomic state

Use your answers from the previous two questions to determine which autonomic state you were in when you were triggered. You might write or say to yourself: '*When my boss ignored me, I started to feel tired and foggy. I had the urge to hide away from the world and my thoughts had an "I can't" flavour to them. This is normally what happens when I'm in the shutdown state.*'

4. Finally, get to the root of your emotional trigger by asking yourself the following questions:

- 'When, in my life, have I experienced something like this before?'

- 'What does it remind me of? Are the feelings familiar?'

- 'What thoughts come with the emotions?'

- 'Is there a specific event from my childhood that stirred up similar emotions?'

Write down your answers to these so that next time you notice yourself in a dysregulated state and are trying to identify your trigger, you can compare and start to notice if there's a pattern.

3.
WAYS TO HEAL YOUR NERVOUS SYSTEM: GLIMMERS

Now that we've got a full understanding of our nervous system and how to identify our triggers, which cause fight-or-flight and shutdown states, we can look at how to heal our nervous systems in both the short term and long term.

As we go through life, engaging with the world, there are inevitably moments when we will feel safe and settled, and others in which we will feel triggered and uneasy. You may feel calm and regulated when you are relaxing in the bath or having dinner with your family, then find yourself in survival mode when you are stuck in traffic, in conflict with a mate, or about to give a presentation at work.

Small detours away from regulation and into dysregulation are normal and to be expected. Dipping into fight-or-flight or shutdown is perfectly healthy so long as you can quickly bounce back to the safe-and-social state after the stressful experience is over. This is what we call having a *resilient* nervous system. It's the ability to flexibly move in and out of different nervous system states without getting stuck. A resilient nervous system, which can quickly bounce back to a state of calm after an uncomfortable experience, is the foundation for reclaiming our authentic selves and is how we invite more joy, connection and creativity into our lives.

WE BECOME RESILIENT WHEN WE HAVE A HEALTHY NERVOUS SYSTEM THAT CAN BOUNCE BACK AFTER A STRESSFUL EXPERIENCE.

Suppose you see a road traffic accident on your morning commute. You might experience a little spike in fight-or-flight energy and feel anxious or uneasy. If your nervous system is resilient enough, you will return to a calm and regulated state by the time you arrive at work. However, if you have an inflex-ible system you might stay in fight-or-flight mode for the rest of the day. Your system might get stuck on high alert, and you could find yourself snapping at your colleagues or panicking about every email that comes through.

If you have experienced trauma or a lot of stress in your life, you are more likely to have an inflexible system that gets stuck in intense or lengthy periods of fight-or-flight or shutdown. Our nervous systems are shaped by our personal histories and continue to be shaped by our day-to-day experiences. If you grew up in a chaotic home, for example, where unpredict-ability and fear were the norm, you will likely have an altered nervous system that is hypersensitive to threats. You may regularly flip-flop between fight-or-flight and shutdown, and find it difficult to make your way home to a calm and regulated state. Even in the absence of adverse childhood experiences or major trauma, chronic stress and the lack of control that goes with it, can be enough to make our nervous systems overly reactive and inflexible.

Before I trained to be a therapist, I worked in the media industry. I began my career in magazine publishing and ended up at a creative agency, where I managed marketing campaigns for various brands. I enjoyed my work, but I spent most of my career stuck in a dysregulated state of fight-or-flight or shutdown. I was so fearful of failing or being judged that quite small daily things could set off my threat response – too many unread emails, a blunt message from my boss, a small mistake on a document for a client.

I didn't know anything about the nervous system then but looking back I can see that I didn't have a very resilient system – I was overly sensitive to harmless triggers and I found it difficult to recover from life's daily stressors. I would habitually get stuck in survival mode, sometimes for weeks at a time.

At times I would be in a permanent state of fight-or-flight, where I would 'over-function' (I like to call this my 'must do everything now' mode). I would work long hours, over-prepare for everything and struggle to delegate (*it's quicker if I just do it!*). Everything felt urgent and I found it almost impossible to switch off and relax in the evening without a glass of wine.

At other times, I would get stuck in a shutdown state, floating through the days with little awareness. In this mode, I would 'under-function' (I like to call this my 'I just can't' mode). I would be quiet in meetings, stay under the radar, miss opportunities and avoid any kind of situation where I needed to be assertive. I could stay in shutdown mode long after I got home from work, feeling unmotivated and too tired to do anything.

I used to confuse fight-or-flight mode for having energy and shutdown mode for laziness, but I can now see that I was dysregulated. As is the case for many of my clients, and possibly for you, my dysregulation wasn't just a result of my job, it was also the result of many decades of unprocessed stress.

Once I learned about the nervous system, I began incorporating my glimmers – the experiences and resources that made me feel safe and settled – into my daily routine. Over time, the stressful moments became just that: moments, with a beginning, middle and end. I also started processing my emotional triggers with my therapist, and I eventually noticed I was spending the majority of my time in a regulated state, where I felt happy, at ease and comfortable in my own skin. Regulation became my new normal.

DYSREGULATION CAN BE THE RESULT OF MANY DECADES OF UNPROCESSED STRESS.

The reassuring and hopeful news is that an inflexible nervous system is not a life sentence. We can *heal* our nervous system and 'retrain' it to spend more time in a safe-and-social state, where we can be our optimal selves. That is what this chapter is all about.

If we want to move though life with more ease, connection and happiness, we need a resilient nervous system – one that can easily return to regulation after experiencing stress.

Glimmers Can Fall Into Two Categories

1 **Self-regulating glimmers:**

These are the things you do on your own to bring yourself into regulation. For example, reading, creating, walking in nature, yoga or a bath.

2 **Co-regulating glimmers:**

These are the things you do with others to come into regulation. For example, laughing with a friend, talking to a therapist, having a deep conversation with your partner or cuddling a pet.

By paying mindful attention to the people, places and experiences that regulate your nervous system, and incorporating them into your daily routine, you can reshape your system away from habitual patterns of fight-or-flight and shutdown. In other words, we identify our 'glimmers'.

HOW TO FIND YOUR GLIMMERS

Glimmers have the opposite effect of triggers. Rather than triggering the nervous system's survival responses, glimmers incite a sense of calm and relaxation. They return us to a state of homeostasis, where our system is balanced and regulated. It sometimes takes a bit of work to notice our glimmers. Our nervous systems are conditioned to look for threats rather than for moments of safety, and the sensations we feel when we are regulated can also be more subtle than those in fight-or-flight and shutdown. We need to pay conscious attention to what makes us feel regulated.

GLIMMERS INCITE A SENSE OF CALM
AND RELAXATION.

EXERCISE: CREATE YOUR GLIMMERS GAMEPLAN

Psychological and physical well-being are best served when we actively participate in regulating practices each and every day. But when we're feeling anxious or disconnected, it can be really difficult to remember our glimmers, and we can forget the positive actions we can take to soothe ourselves. Yet it's at these low points that we need our glimmers the most!

Over the next few days, pay attention to what makes your system feel at ease and make a list of your glimmers. What activities make you feel nourished and relaxed? Who makes you feel safe and accepted? Which places make you feel happy and at peace?

Then gather your glimmers in one place so that you can refer to them next time you feel dysregulated. I have mine saved as a pinned note on my phone, but you might want to write them in your notebook, illustrate them in a journal or create a collage or Pinterest board. Just make sure they are accessible so that you can easily reach for them when you system becomes dysregulated.

If you are looking for some inspiration, here are some common examples of glimmers:

Being in nature

Breathing exercises

Yoga

Connecting with others

Mindfulness

Music

Journaling

Kissing

Baths

Art/creating

Certain TV/movies

Dancing

Massage

Laughing

Swimming

Hugs

Singing

Organising

Flirting

Favourite foods

Playing

Reading

Time alone

Exercising

Meditating

Cooking

Gardening

Time with animals

Walking

THE GOLDILOCKS PRINCIPLE

Taking our glimmers one step further, to regulate our nervous system, it's important to develop the capacity to recognise which nervous system state we are in and to respond *effectively*. In other words, different states will require different types of glimmers.

A really helpful way to think about this is by applying the 'Goldilocks Principle'. Through doing this, we begin to recognise when we are feeling either 'too hot' in fight-or-flight mode (anxious, overwhelmed, irritable or panicky) or 'too cold' in shutdown mode (depressed, numb, tired and withdrawn).

When we are 'too hot', we generally need glimmers that are aimed at discharging energy in the body and move us towards relaxation, like running, dancing, singing, organising or playing. When we are 'too cold', we usually need regulating practices that are aimed towards gently mobilising and re-energising the body, like a hot bath/shower, a walk, a phone call with a friend, or sitting in a place where there are people and activity.

When I'm in shutdown state ('too cold'), the thought of going for a run can feel impossible. In fact, just putting on my trainers can feel like a mountain to climb. But having a hot shower, texting my friend or even just listening to my 'running' playlist all feel more achievable. These actions can ease me out of my collapsed state and gently re-energise me. However, when I am in fight-or-flight mode ('too hot') and I feel frantic or on-edge, going for a run can be exactly what I need to discharge my energy and relax my system.

Glimmers should be aimed towards either relaxing or re-energising the system, depending on what is needed to feel 'just right'. Being able to recognise which autonomic state you're in and respond with the correct glimmer for *you* is an incredible life skill and an essential step on the road to reconnecting with your true self. Next time you need to use one of your glimmers, practise firstly identifying which state you're in and then choosing one of your glimmers accordingly. It'll take time to develop this skill, but it truly is a tool that will transform how you respond and feel every day.

Everyday glimmers

When our nervous systems have become 'stuck' in a fight-or-flight or shutdown state, we need to do daily work to heal our systems. The good news is the positive effects of glimmers are cumulative. So, each time we soothe our system and restore a state of calm, we are building new pathways to relaxation and developing more resilience and flexibility in our system.

The most powerful glimmers to engage in regularly, and to integrate into your daily life, are what I like to call the six healing powerhouses: movement, breath, co-regulation, nature, play and awe.

> THE GOAL ISN'T TO BE IN A ZEN-LIKE STATE OF REGULATION ALL THE TIME – WE NEED OUR THREAT RESPONSES TO KEEP US ALIVE.

The goal isn't to be in a zen-like state of regulation all the time – we need our threat responses to keep us alive. In fact, it's a normal human experience to move through different autonomic states many times a day. It's only when we move out of safety and can't find our way back to regulation that we suffer physically and emotionally.

Before we dive into the six healing powerhouses, I want to paint a picture of what life could look like for you once you have healed your nervous system and developed more resilience:

- Life's daily stressors become much more manageable and you no longer 'sweat the small stuff'. When you spill your coffee or miss your train, you can remain calm and regulated, and 'go with the flow' (instead of spinning-out and feeling anxious or detached for hours or days on end).
- If something does dysregulate your system, and you find yourself in fight, flight or shutdown mode, you can quickly recover and return to your baseline once the stressful situation has passed. (Remember, we're not trying to be regulated all the time. We will inevitably encounter events that are stressful enough to dysregulate our system.)
- The regulated safe-and-social state will become your new normal and the world will feel like a much more inviting place to live. You will spend most of your time feeling present, calm and connected, and in both your personal and professional life you will feel more comfortable being your authentic self.

THE 6 HEALING POWERHOUSES

1. Movement

We all know that exercise is good for our overall physical health, but it's also a powerful way to rebalance the nervous

6 Healing Powerhouses

Movement

Breath

Nature

Co-regulation

Play

Awe

system. When it comes to exercise for self-regulation, we each need to find the right way to move, depending on our nervous system's state.

As I mentioned earlier, when you are in fight-or-flight mode, your mind and body are ready for action – tight jaw, gripping hands, tense muscles. If you are prone to feeling like this in your daily life then you might be more drawn to high-intensity exercise, as a way to discharge your energy and move you towards a state of relaxation. I know when I've had a stressful day or I'm feeling particularly anxious, I can feel a lot calmer after I've sweated it out at a spin class or on a run.

If you tend towards shutdown mode, where you feel flat in mood and low in energy, you may be more drawn to lighter exercise like walking or yoga. This type of exercise *gently* re-energises us. When I'm in a shutdown state and I feel collapsed and unmotivated, even a short walk to the shops can 'wake up' my system and bring my body closer to a state of balance.

However, it's important to understand that there is no one-size-fits-all rule when it comes to exercise as a way to regulate our nervous system. In fact, the movement we are drawn to might not even be what's best for regulating our system. If you find yourself in a shutdown state and you're drawn to a gentle yoga practice, you may actually find that getting outside and going for a run is more energising for you and creates a feeling of more balance. Alternatively, if you find yourself in a fight-or-flight state and you're drawn to high-intensity exercise to discharge your stress, you might in fact find that a gentle walk on the beach is a more effective way to come back to your baseline.

Using movement to regulate your nervous system requires mind-body awareness and always begins with recognising which state your nervous system is in, then responding effectively. This, of course, takes some trial and error, but you will likely soon discover that even 10 minutes of the *right* type of movement can significantly reduce anxiety or improve your energy levels.

Regardless of which type of movement you choose for self-regulation, it's important that you maintain some awareness *as you move*. This means placing all of your attention (or as much as you can) on the soothing or energising benefit of the movement. Being mindful in moments of movement really allows the positive effects to land in our mind-body, rather than letting it pass us by. There have been plenty of times when I have gone for a run and spent the whole time thinking through my to-do list, paying very little attention to how my body is feeling. I used to feel this was a good use of time (hey, I'm multitasking!), but when I started to run in a more mindful way, paying attention to how the energy in my body was changing, I always ended up feeling more relaxed and regulated by the time I got home.

EXERCISE: SHAKE IT OFF

It sounds very woo-woo and weird but shaking the body can be a powerful way to discharge stress and rebalance the nervous system. In his book *Waking the Tiger: Healing Trauma*, Dr Peter A. Levine notes that animals can be observed shaking or vibrating after a stressful experience to release tension, burn excess adrenaline and regulate their nervous system. All mammals do it, except for us, because we've learned to control it.

The practice is simple: stand hip-width apart, soften your knees and let your body feel loose like a rag doll. Then begin shaking, moving or bouncing in whatever way your body feels like for a few minutes. Really good music can help!

It may sound totally bonkers, and you will undoubtedly feel odd the first time you do it, but shaking is a quick and simple technique that signals to your body that the stressful situation has passed and you're now safe to relax.

2. Breath

The breath is one of the quickest and easiest ways to move our system into a regulated state. Breath is controlled by the autonomic nervous system, and, while it's an automatic process, it's also one that we can intentionally control. We can't tell our heart to beat slower or our adrenal glands to release less adrenaline, but we can deepen and slow our breath, and gently guide our system towards a calm and resting state.

When our mind-body thinks we're under threat, we don't take full, deep and steady breaths. In fight-or-flight, our breath tends to be short, sharp and fast. In shutdown, our breath tends to be flat, shallow and quiet. When we take full, slow and deep breaths, we are able to switch our physiology from dysregulated to regulated, from a felt-sense of danger to a felt-sense of safety. As with anything that regulates the system, this tells the nervous system that the threat has passed, and you are now safe.

DEEPENING AND SLOWING OUR BREATH CAN GENTLY GUIDE OUR SYSTEM TOWARDS A CALM AND RESTING STATE.

EXERCISE: A DEEP SIGH

We tend to associate a deep sigh with the expression of frustration, despair or relief, but sighing also serves as a type of reset button for our nervous system. When we exhale for longer than we inhale, we release tension and prompt the body to 'switch off' survival mode (fight, flight or shutdown) and 'switch on' safe-and-social mode.

A deep sigh is simple and perfect for when you feel your emotions are about to take off on a rollercoaster ride:

1. Sit in a comfortable position with your neck and shoulders relaxed.

2. Keeping your mouth closed, inhale slowly through your nostrils for four seconds.

3. Exhale through your mouth or nose for six seconds (the idea is that your exhale should be longer than your inhale).

4. Keep your breath slow and steady while breathing out.

EXERCISE: BOX BREATHING

Box breathing (also known as square breathing) is one of my favourite techniques for calming anxiety. It's a powerful relaxation technique that aims to return breathing to its normal rhythm:

1. Breathe in through your nose while slowly counting to four. Feel the air enter your lungs.

2. Hold your breath inside while counting slowly to four. Try not to clamp your mouth or nose shut. Simply avoid inhaling or exhaling for four seconds.

3. Begin to slowly exhale for four seconds.

4. Pause for four seconds. Then repeat the steps at least four times.

You should find that after a handful of rounds of box breathing, your nervous system has returned to a more regulated state.

3. Co-Regulation

When we are emotionally distressed and dysregulated, having someone there with us – whether it's a friend, partner or family member – can make soothing our nervous system a lot easier. As mentioned earlier, this practice is called co-regulation – it's the wonderful process of using another person's calm nervous system to regulate our own. It's why when you are anxious or upset, and someone you love sits with you or gives you a hug, you can suddenly feel calm and settled.

Humans are social animals. From the moment we are born we need to feel safe in our relationships with others, and this need lasts until the moment we die. We may live in a culture where self-sufficiency is congratulated and dependency is discouraged, but our nervous systems never stop needing, and longing for, safe and dependable relationships. As Deb Dana puts it, 'Co-regulation is essential; first for survival and then for living a life of well-being'.

Co-regulation is not the same as merely being in the presence of other people. Being in the presence of a calm and regulated person is soothing because it sends the message to our nervous system that we are no longer in danger and it's safe to relax.

IF WE WANT OUR PHYSIOLOGY TO CALM DOWN, WE NEED TO FEEL TRULY SEEN AND HEARD BY A PERSON WHO IS THEMSELVES REGULATED.

Conversely, being in the presence of a dysregulated person, who is in a state of fight-or-flight, or shutdown, can send the message to our nervous system that something threatening is in the vicinity and we should be on high alert. When others are regulated, we can become regulated. When others are dysregulated, we can become dysregulated. We can effectively 'mirror' the autonomic state of the people around us.

If we want to feel the incredible benefits of co-regulation, we also need to regulate with the right people. Start paying attention to how your nervous system feels in the presence of others. Do you regularly go from feeling chilled-out to anxious and on-edge when you are with a certain family member? Do you always end-up feeling low and self-critical after spending time with a particular friend?

As you heal and grow your capacity for regulation, you can learn to notice which relationships drain you and which nourish you. The goal is to spend more time with the people in your life that bring you a feeling of being safe and welcome. Remember, the quality of your relationships has much more impact on your well-being than the quantity.

* * *

For some ideas on co-regulating glimmers, see page 51.

Co-regulating with animals

Co-regulation isn't just reserved for our relationships with humans. We can also derive a lot of comfort from other mammals like dogs, cats or horses. Relationships with animals can offer less complicated connections than with humans, and can predictably bring us into a safe-and-social state. One of the best parts about needing to move my private practice online during the pandemic was getting to meet some of my clients' pets. I could feel their nervous systems relax when they stroked their dog or when their cat came and sat on their lap. They would become more present, open and calm.

4. Awe

We feel awe when we encounter something with qualities so extraordinary it seems incomprehensible: the birth of a child; the vast expanse of a star-filled sky; a mind-blowing concert.

Awe is a feeling of wonder that makes you feel both small and connected to something larger than yourself. We often experience awe when we feel touched by the beauty of nature, art, music or spirituality. These goosebump-inducing moments shift our attention away from ourselves, trigger a deep sense of appreciation and change our perception or understanding of things.

Moments of awe are associated with the safe-and-social state, and have the ability to move our nervous system from a dysregulated state, where we feel anxious, angry or hopeless, to

4 Ways to Experience More Awe

1. Go out into nature and really pay attention to your environment (that might mean putting your phone away!). Slow down and try looking for things you've never seen before and listening to sounds you might not normally hear when you are rushing around with headphones in.

2. Novelty can be a big part of awe so try visiting a new place, listening to a different type of music or even just taking a different route and noticing your surroundings.

3. Part of awe involves embracing uncertainty and ambiguity. Try engaging with the world with an open-mind and let go of the need to understand or explain moments of beauty. When we feel awe, it's best to simply stand back and admire.

4. Awe can also come from connecting with impressive people and stories. Try listening to an inspiring speech or reading a story about an act of great courage. Fully appreciating the value of others can help us see humanity through a more positive and hopeful lens.

a more regulated state, where we feel happy, present and at ease. Research has found that awe may also protect our health, make us more generous, decrease materialism, and make us feel more connected to other people and humanity.

The good news is that you don't need to visit the Taj Mahal or climb to the summit of Mount Everest to reap the many benefits of awe. Awe can also be found in everyday experiences: watching a beautiful sunset, listening to powerful music, or noticing the intricate pattern on the wings of a butterfly.

5. Nature

The need for nature is in our wiring. Intuitively, most of us feel that spending time in nature is good for our well-being, but science now confirms it: nature regulates the autonomic nervous system. We now know that being in a natural environment reduces the fight-or-flight response, evokes a feeling of safety, and can bring us back into a regulated state following a stressful experience.

Time in nature can be a hugely nourishing and restorative experience, but as with anything that helps soothe our nervous system, our levels of awareness and 'connectedness' to the experience greatly impacts the positive benefits. Connectedness with nature goes beyond simply *being in* nature; it's about actively engaging with nature through our senses and emotions.

Pacing through your local park while you reply to emails isn't going to have the same calming effect on your nervous system as a gentle stroll, where you listen to birdsong and reflect on the beauty of the trees. It is the *quality*, not quantity, of our time spent in nature that contributes to its positive impact on

3 Ways You Can Develop Your Own 'Nature-Connectedness'

1 Nature isn't just found in rural areas. Even in cities where nature can be harder to find, you can experience the regulating effects of nature if you tune in and stay present in your surroundings. Notice the changing seasons, listen out for birdsong, or reflect on the beauty of the moving clouds. All of these things can help soothe your nervous system and send a signal to your brain that everything is all right.

2 You don't always need to leave the house to connect with nature. Caring for indoor plants can be deeply nourishing or simply having flowers in a room can invite moments of joy. Surprisingly, research has even found that experiencing 'technological nature' is better than no nature, which means watching a nature documentary, or looking at a screensaver of a landscape, might send the message to your mind-body that it's safe to relax.

3 A powerful way to improve your connection to nature is to combine nature with creativity. Take photos, write, draw or paint pictures, or incorporate foraged materials into your crafting. Expressing the beauty of nature creatively can be restorative and uplifting, and deepen your appreciation of the world around you.

our nervous system and well-being, though, for many of us, quality time in nature may not be as easy as it sounds.

6. Play

In our culture, where our self-worth is tied to our productivity, making time for play is rare. In fact, by the time we reach adulthood, we can convince ourselves that being playful is a time-consuming luxury we can no longer afford. Yet, research consistently shows us that adult play is an important part of well-being and can have a significant impact on the health of our nervous system.

Play is considered a purposeless activity that brings about joy and pleasure. Play might involve dancing, games, singing, expressing yourself through painting, colouring or making music. It can be so enjoyable that we become engrossed in the activity and lose sense of time with a child-like abandon. Play is an act that should be engaged in for its own sake; not for the purpose of winning or improving yourself. That means going on a bike ride for the fun of it, not because you're trying to burn calories.

ADULT PLAY CAN HAVE A SIGNIFICANT IMPACT ON THE HEALTH OF OUR NERVOUS SYSTEM.

Play can reshape our nervous system and strengthen our ability to flexibly move between different nervous system states, particularly when the activity is social. When we play a board game with our mates or have a snowball fight with our partner, our nervous system can shift in and out of the fight-or-flight and safe-and-social states. Fight-or-flight can get activated in moments of excitement or pretend danger, and the safe-and-social state can get activated in the moments that are more tender or calm. In other words, play is healing because it is a way to activate the fight-or-flight response in a safe environment. When there is no real threat, and the activity is fun, play 'retrains' our nervous system to better tolerate, and recover from, fight-or-flight mode – the essence of autonomic resilience.

We all have the ability to be playful people, but sometimes our inner critic can be a barrier. That negative voice inside your head might tell you that play is silly, unproductive or a complete waste of time. To embrace more playful parts of yourself, try exploring adult versions of the playful activities that brought you joy as a child. If you liked Play-Doh, maybe you could take a sculpture class, or if you loved dressing-up maybe you could experiment with make-up tutorials on YouTube. Remember, play isn't about the result, it's about doing something for the sheer delight of doing it.

* * *

EXERCISE: INCORPORATING GLIMMERS INTO YOUR EVERYDAY LIFE

Revisit the list of personal glimmers you've made after the exercise on page 50. Check to see if:

1. You have a type of glimmer from each of the six powerhouses. If you don't, see if you can choose one that you'd like.

2. Of these, pick one which you can introduce into your daily life this week.

3. See how bringing this regular glimmer into your life starts to soothe your nervous system after a while. When you feel ready, choose another glimmer from one of the other powerhouses.

4. The aim is to try and incorporate at least one glimmer from each of the healing powerhouses.

PART 2

BREAKING DOWN BARRIERS TO BEING YOUR TRUE SELF

4.
PEOPLE-PLEASING

Now that we're equipped with a thorough understanding of our nervous system, we're ready to start looking at the coping strategies we've developed that might be preventing us from being our true selves. These are the ways we *think* help us feel safe, when instead they're acting as further barriers to us feeling regulated and comfortable in our own skin. Let's start with one of the most common self-defeating mechanisms: people-pleasing.

On the face of it, it might seem like people-pleasing is all about being caring, thoughtful or wanting other people to be happy, but it's a pattern of behaviour that unfortunately comes with a lot of problems. If you're a people-pleaser, you may struggle to say what you want, or you don't like to disagree with others. You might find yourself apologising when it's not your fault or saying yes to things when, really, you want to say no. At the centre of this is a hard truth: when we are people-pleasing, we aren't just *being nice*; we are trying to avoid the discomfort of being disliked.

I used to be a people-pleaser. On the surface, I appeared easy-going and flexible, but underneath my 'cool girl' persona

I was terrified of going against the grain or making people unhappy. I worried that if I expressed what I needed, I would appear pushy, rude or selfish, so I mirrored other people's opinions: *'You want the bigger room? Sure, no problem'*; *'Need to borrow some money? Of course, how much do you need?'*

I thought abandoning my boundaries was the best way to avoid conflict and to gain approval. To make things worse, I wasn't even consciously aware that I was doing it most of the time.

> WHEN WE ARE PEOPLE-PLEASING,
> WE AREN'T JUST BEING NICE; WE ARE
> TRYING TO AVOID THE DISCOMFORT
> OF BEING DISLIKED.

My preoccupation with everyone else's happiness was so consuming that, at times, I even lost sight of my own likes and dislikes. I would let other people make decisions on where we should go, what we should do, and even what we should eat. This wasn't because I was laid-back or selfless, but instead because the thought of making a decision that disappointed or inconvenienced someone else made me feel anxious. Despite this, instead of telling someone what I wanted, it felt safer to disregard my own preferences and focus on everyone else's. I was so busy tuning in to what everyone else needed that I forgot to tune in to myself and, some days, I felt like I didn't even have my own identity.

COMMON SIGNS OF PEOPLE-PLEASING:

- You say 'yes' to things you don't really want to do

- You feel guilty if you put yourself first

- You automatically feel at fault if someone is angry with you

- You take the blame for things that aren't your responsibility

- You feel responsible for making everyone happy so you overthink every interaction, worrying that you might have upset someone

- You have a preoccupation with what others think about you

- You need a lot of approval and praise, and have crashing lows when you receive feedback or criticism

- You have difficulty expressing your own needs, feelings and boundaries

- You are overly concerned with how others are feeling

- You have difficulty feeling anger towards other people

- You are overly flexible and always want to appear helpful

- You avoid conflict and mirror other people's opinions

- You shape-shift into being whatever you think different people need you to be and, as a result, feel like you have no identity

- You are exhausted by having to maintain the appearance of being OK all the time, and you struggle to be vulnerable for fear of being rejected or disliked

HELPING OTHERS, LOSING YOURSELF

I used to think that a major benefit of my people-pleasing was that I could make friends with anyone. I was very proud of my ability to read other people and adjust myself to fit into any social situation. But here's the kicker: shape-shifting to fit in with other people doesn't lead to great friends and a deep sense of belonging; it makes us feel lonely. Ironically, being a social chameleon, and adjusting our personality to be the version of ourselves that we think will gain the most approval, actually distances us from other people. Rather than lead us to a sense of connection, it makes us feel unseen and unknown, because we're never showing people who we really are.

> WHEN WE SHAPE-SHIFT TO FIT IN WITH OTHER PEOPLE IT DOESN'T LEAD TO DEEP RELATIONSHIPS OR BELONGING, IT MAKES US FEEL LONELY.

We may even be left feeling resentful in our relationships and wonder why nobody is asking us how we are doing or what we want. By constantly putting everyone else first, it's unlikely we're getting our needs met by others and our relationships can become one-sided. We might even end up becoming a 'martyr' and see others as being demanding or selfish. It's easy for a feeling of overwhelm to develop when we're surrounded by people who depend on us and, over time, this can lead to resentment.

A very common area of life where people please is with friendships. A client of mine was constantly prioritising their friends' needs over their own. They'd always say OK to travelling across London to see their friend, or inconvenience themselves in other ways, like spending more money than they wanted to going to a restaurant, or sacrifice their self-care time to suit their friend's schedule. In conversations, too, this client would always ask their friends, '*what's going on with you?*' but would quickly deflect the conversation away from themselves. Unfortunately, this behaviour led to resentment, as their friends became conditioned to the idea that my client either didn't have opinions, or didn't want to talk about themselves. The dynamic became one sided, and my client started to feel unseen and resented doing things they never truly wanted to do.

If you feel like you don't get any or enough attention in your relationships, it doesn't necessarily mean you have surrounded yourself with self-absorbed narcissists (although sometimes it does!). It may be that you, too, have spent so long hyper-focusing on others and deflecting conversations away from yourself, that you have effectively taught people that you don't want or need the focus to ever be on you.

I find it helpful to think of people-pleasing as an invisible shield that we carry around with us in the hope that it will protect us from being disliked or rejected. We unconsciously hope that if we move through life putting everyone's needs ahead of our own, we will be safe and loved. The reality is that people-pleasing is a heavy piece of armour with some high costs: it makes us feel anxious and resentful; it prevents us from living authentically; and it interferes with our ability to connect with people on a deep level.

The hard thing is that after years of people pleasing in this way, you can lose sight of what you think and how you feel. You get to the point where you don't know what you need or want. There is, however, a path out of people-pleasing, and part of breaking the people-pleasing pattern is to stop over-focusing on how everyone else feels, and start listening to our own true wants, needs and desires. When we can release the grip on our need to please, many of us can finally ask ourselves about our own dreams: *'What do I want out of life? Out of my career? Out of my relationships? Out of my free time?'* This is how we journey back to who we really are and own our full identity.

THE SCIENCE BEHIND OUR NEED TO PLEASE

In earlier chapters we looked at the fight-or-flight and shut-down responses, which are automatic responses to danger in all human beings. We saw how fight-or-flight is triggered when we respond to something stressful by being angry or by launching into hyper-activity, whereas the shutdown response is triggered when we respond to stress by numbing-out or withdrawing. But another specific way in which humans can respond to some-thing stressful is to go into 'fawn' mode – a survival response at the core of people-pleasing behaviour.

The 'fawn' response is triggered when we respond to a threat by trying to be pleasing, nice or helpful. If you think

Reminders for Recovering People-Pleasers

All healthy relationships have boundaries

It's not your job to make everyone happy

Saying 'yes' when you want to say 'no' leads to resentment

It's okay if your boundaries disappoint people

It's not selfish to choose things that preserve your well-being your boss is mad at you or you sense an argument brewing with a friend, you may default to fawn mode and start pleasing, appeasing and possibly complimenting the other person so that things don't escalate. Fawning is all about making other people happy and comfortable in order to feel safe and avoid being hurt. Unlike fight-or-flight or shutdown, which are innate and automatic stress responses in all humans, the fawn response is a *learned* behaviour. But once it has been learned, it can become our go-to way of trying to feel safe.

The fawn response was first coined by therapist Pete Walker to describe how some people will please and flatter others in order to gain love and avoid potential problems. Walker says, 'Fawn types seek safety by merging with the wishes, needs and demands of others. They act as if they believe that the price of admission into any relationship is the forfeiture of all their needs, rights, preferences and boundaries.'

The people-pleasing fawn response is often learned in our early years. When you were a child, you may have discovered that when something stressful or dangerous was happening in your relationships, fighting, running or dissociating from it didn't work to keep you safe or out of trouble, but fawning did. Perhaps you noticed that when you asked for help, your father would become angry but when you were useful or amenable, you could diffuse his rage. Or you may have learned that expressing your preferences or opinions made your mother withdraw from you, but when you were agreeable and sweet, you received some positive attention. Many people-pleasers grew up in environ-ments where carefully monitoring other people's moods was a pathway to safety.

The Root Causes of Fawning as a Survival Response Tend to Fall Into Two Categories

1 **You learned it was important to please people:** Many people-pleasers started out as parent-pleasers. Perhaps you were excessively praised for being 'good' and 'kind' to the point where your identity became tied up with being easy-going, thoughtful or considerate. You may have been given the label in your family as the 'kind' one, the 'thoughtful' one, or the 'mediator'. In an attempt to please your parents and maintain a sense of connection and belonging, you may have desperately tried to live up to your label, perhaps denying your true self in the process.

2 **You learned it was important to not displease people:** Some children are punished, silenced or ignored when they try to assert their needs and, as a result, learn to barely show themselves. You may have learned from a young age that it doesn't feel OK or safe to express yourself authentically so you hid behind a helpful persona to avoid any drama. You may have stopped having any preferences or boundaries that might have angered your parents, or learned to minimise any needs that might have inconvenienced them.

The result of both of these scenarios on the previous page is the internalisation of the idea that being loved is dependent on how 'good' we are, and that making other people happy is how we can feel safe and secure in relationships. Unfortunately, when we have a tendency to please our way towards love and security, we lose touch with our sense of self and can struggle to feel truly seen or known in our relationships.

EXERCISE: AM I PEOPLE-PLEASING OR AM I JUST BEING KIND?

When I talk about people-pleasing I often get asked, 'How do I know if I'm people-pleasing or just being kind?' The answer can usually be found by identifying the *intention* behind your behaviour, because with people-pleasing behaviours there are always hidden fears or motivations lurking in the background. You might agree with someone because you are trying to seek approval or you might be extra flexible because you are trying to avoid conflict.

Here are two questions you can ask yourself to help you tell the difference:

Question 1: 'If I don't do ____, what am I afraid will happen?'

People-pleasing isn't about wanting to be nice. It's about trying to organise the reactions of other people to avoid criticism, conflict, judgement or rejection. If you are people-pleasing, the answer to the above question might sound something like: *'they will be mad at me'; 'they will think I'm selfish'; 'they won't like me any more'; 'they won't ask me again'.*

Question 2: 'If I do ____, what benefit do I receive?'

The motivation to please others can sometimes be a form of altruism – we might genuinely want to be kind or want other people to have the help they need. In other cases, people-pleasing is a way of receiving external validation or feeling safe. If you are people-pleasing, the answer to this question might sound something like: *'I will be complimented'*; *'I will be praised'*; *'I will be appreciated'*; *'I will be loved'*.

PEOPLE-PLEASING AT WORK

Before we look at how to tackle people-pleasing, it's worth focusing on one of the hardest places to break the people-pleasing: the workplace. In many ways, our culture rewards people-pleasing behaviours at work, but whether you are an intern or a CEO, the cost of people-pleasing in your career can be high.

In my clinical practice as a therapist, I see people every day who are permanently stressed and on the verge of burnout because they are so focused on proving their worth or not rocking the boat at work. If you're a people-pleaser, you might often over-extend yourself by saying 'yes' to everything or by offering help to everyone, regardless of your own workload or capacity. You tend to take on more work than you can comfortably manage in a bid to feel secure, liked and valued, but wind up feeling unappreciated, anxious, and resentful. What's more, as a people-pleaser you'll typically want to be liked and respected but you tend to give up your power and can get steamrolled by others, which contrarily leads to a lack of respect.

Here are some examples of how people-pleasing behaviours can show up in your career, whether you are employed or you are self-employed:

THE PEOPLE-PLEASING FAWN RESPONSE WHEN YOU ARE EMPLOYED MIGHT LOOK LIKE:

- Taking on additional work and solving other people's problems in an attempt to win favour

- Difficulty delegating

- Not taking allocated holiday time

- Attending unnecessary meetings because you don't want to disappoint people

- Running your decisions past other people to make sure nobody disagrees with your choices

- Taking on duties that aren't even part of your job description

- Failing to hold people accountable out of a desire to be popular

- Volunteering for unpopular projects to show that you are helpful

- Remaining quiet in group settings in order to maintain harmony

- Responding to every request for support, even if it interrupts your own work

THE PEOPLE-PLEASING FAWN RESPONSE WHEN YOU ARE SELF-EMPLOYED MIGHT LOOK LIKE:

- Doing too much work for free

- Offering discounts without being asked

- Saying yes to tasks you can't complete

- Working all the time without breaks

- Taking on more than you can comfortably manage because you don't want to disappoint people

- Feeling disconnected from your true voice because you are afraid of offending people

- Only charging what you think people can afford, rather than what you are worth

- Overcommitting because you can't say 'no', then feeling stressed, overwhelmed or incompetent

Dissatisfied at work

If you're a people-pleaser, you may hope, sometimes unconsciously, that your hard work and generosity will be rewarded, perhaps with a pay rise, promotion or even just some words of appreciation. But when this doesn't happen, the disappointment can be gut-wrenching. You feel let down, unappreciated and taken for granted. But rather than viewing these feelings as a signal to introduce some boundaries or to find a better work-life balance, you work harder, stay later and please more, in the hope that your efforts will someday be noticed and rewarded. Eventually, when you notice that everyone else is only doing what their job demands and nothing more, you start to simmer with anger and resentment: *'She can't stay late tonight because she has plans? I always stay late to make sure everything is done!'*; or *'I can't believe nobody is going to volunteer to work on this extra project! I always put myself forward; isn't it someone else's turn for a change?'*

The problem with the unspoken transaction of people-pleasing is that the other people involved never signed up for this reciprocal arrangement in the first place. Over-giving in the hope that it will win you favour or yield results will only lead to frustration and resentment when you don't get repaid or rewarded for your efforts. What's more, over-giving effectively trains your employers and colleagues to lean on you. The more you appear to handle, the more you will be expected to handle. If you always reply to emails late at night, or you are always the one to cover other people's work when they are sick, you aren't signing an unspoken contract where colleagues will over-give back to you in return. Far from it. You are conditioning people into expecting you to always be the over-accommodating 'yes' person, and you are making a rod for your own back. Flexibility, reliability and helpfulness are excellent traits for an employee but if we want to prevent feeling bitter and resentful, we need to only do what we have the capacity to do, and to do it without any strings attached.

People sometimes compulsively people-please in their careers because their workplace relationships mirror dynamics from their family of origin. Bosses can unconsciously remind us of our parents and hook us back into childhood ways of relating. Maybe your boss has a fault-finding manner that reminds you of your mother, so you over-work and over-please in a bid to avoid criticism. Or perhaps you compulsively please your manager because you want the recognition you never received from your father. Until we can recognise that we are inadvertently replaying patterns from the past, we might never feel empowered to stand up for ourselves and break the people-pleasing pattern.

FIND YOUR COMMUNICATION STYLE

No matter what area of life you people-please in most, one of the most powerful ways to liberate ourselves from people-pleasing is to become mindful of how we express our needs and boundaries and to develop a more assertive communication style.

It's a common misconception that assertiveness means being pushy, difficult, rude and disrespectful of other people. But being assertive doesn't have to be any of those things.

BEING ASSERTIVE JUST MEANS VALUING AND COMMUNICATING YOUR NEEDS IN A WAY THAT IS CLEAR AND DIRECT, WHILE STILL RESPECTING OTHERS.

In order to fully grasp what assertive communication is and isn't, it's helpful to understand the four key communication styles: passive; aggressive; passive-aggressive; and assertive. Read through the following styles, and see which resonates with you the most. Each has an animal listed alongside, which I find can be a useful reminder for that style of communicating.

Passive communication (Being like a Turtle)

'I'm OK with whatever you want': Passive communicators are typically quiet and don't seek attention. Turtle-like behaviour includes not expressing feelings or needs in an attempt to prevent being hurt, judged or rejected. This is the communication style normally adopted by people-pleasers. It can look like an inability to say no, acting indifferent during debates or rarely taking a strong stance. Passive communicators act like other people's rights and needs take precedence over their own.

Aggressive communication (Being like a Tiger)

'This is what we're doing': Aggressive communicators frequently express their thoughts and feelings and tend to dominate conversations, often at the expense of others. Tiger-like behaviour is bossy, intimidating, dominating and forceful with a need to control. It can look like being insensitive to the feelings of others (but very sensitive to oneself), interrupting people while they are speaking and being inappropriately honest or direct. Aggressive communicators act like their rights and needs are more important than anyone else's.

Passive-aggressive communication (Being like a Fox)

'I guess we'll do whatever you want to do': Passive-aggressive communicators appear passive on the surface but have more aggressive motivations driving their behaviour. People who develop fox-like communication usually feel powerless and

resentful – they think they don't deserve to speak their minds or they are afraid to express their anger. Passive-aggressive behaviour can look like hurtful teasing disguised as joking, sarcasm or denying there is a problem. Passive-aggressive communicators express their anger by subtly undermining the object of their resentments.

Assertive communication (Being like an Owl)

'I would prefer it if we did this': Assertive communication is the preferred communication style and includes valuing and communicating a boundary or point of view in a way that is clear and direct, while still respecting others. Owl-like communicators firmly advocate for their rights and needs without acting overly aggressive or defensive. It can look like speaking in a calm, empathic and clear tone without interrupting others, being equally respectful to others as to oneself, and expressing preferences honestly and appropriately. Assertive communicators clearly express that both people have rights and needs.

Overcoming people-pleasing and becoming more assertive isn't always easy, particularly if you are shy by nature. One of my clients always struggled between recognising the difference between being assertive and being aggressive. Naturally shy, they would often conflate the two and would think that speaking up to convey a preference or set a boundary was aggressive. They'd assume that if they did that thing, then others would think they're rude. Together, we worked on starting small – for example, for them it was expressing an opinion on what restaurant they went to with their partner – and gradually they began to realise that their friends and family responded well to hearing their opinion. They weren't angry or offended at all. These positive experiences brought my client greater confidence and so they felt better able to articulate more of their opinions. The benefits of speaking up can be life changing. When we're assertive, we ask for what we want, and we talk openly about what we need, and we effectively advocate for ourselves without being pushy. Developing a more assertive communication style can liberate you from resentment, propel your career forward and deepen relationships across all areas of your life.

EXERCISE: ASSERTIVE COMMUNICATION

It takes practice to feel confident enough to stand up for what you believe in, and to tell others truthfully how you're feeling. To get you started, here are some useful phrases/conversation starters that can be jumping-off points for you to communicate your true thoughts:

- *I would prefer it if we did …*

- *I disagree with …*

- *I'm curious about …*

- *I didn't appreciate …*

- *I feel offended by …*

- *Would you mind …*

- *I would prefer not to …*

- *I believe the best way forward is …*

- *I would appreciate it if …*

Dealing with discomfort

Healing from people-pleasing begins with recognising the ways our people-pleasing behaviours have been misguided attempts to receive love and approval. Slowly, with time, we can begin to practise setting boundaries, asserting ourselves, speaking our truth and prioritising our own needs. It isn't easy though. When we've spent a lifetime putting ourselves on the back-burner, it can feel uncomfortable and even scary to start prioritising and pleasing ourselves.

One of the first things people notice when they start to communicate their wants, needs and preferences is a feeling of guilt or fear. You might feel guilty for no longer being as accommodating as you once were, or you might feel afraid that your honesty will hurt someone's feelings or lead to rejection. It's important to remember that just because you *feel* guilty or scared, it doesn't mean that you are doing something 'wrong'. In fact, these uncomfortable feelings are an inevitable part of the process of letting go of people-pleasing, and are what therapists call 'growing pains'. Similar to the way physical growth causes aches and pains in childhood, personal growth can cause emotional discomfort in adulthood. Our challenge is to learn to tolerate the temporary discomfort.

If you've spent your whole life denying your needs to keep other people happy, it will take a bit of time for your nervous system to adjust to the idea that it's safe to communicate honestly and authentically. You may feel anxious if you speak-up about a preference when you would normally say 'I don't mind' or you may feel guilty when you tell someone that you are upset when you would normally say 'I'm fine'. Don't let this discomfort push you back into a space that you're trying to outgrow. Even if you sense someone's disappointment, frustration or sadness, try to resist the urge to 'retract' your boundary or to 'fix' their emotions. Breaking up with people-pleasing means recognising two key things: we have the right to express ourselves authentically; and we are not responsible for managing other people's emotional experiences.

> IT WILL TAKE YOUR NERVOUS SYSTEM TIME TO ADJUST TO THE IDEA THAT IT'S SAFE TO COMMUNICATE HONESTLY AND AUTHENTICALLY.

During these moments of discomfort, it's essential that you look after yourself a little bit more than you might otherwise do. This means making choices that will regulate your nervous system. Check back to Chapter 1, the exercise on page 50, to remind yourself of your glimmers, which can help regulate your system, and soothe your stress with practices that help you feel safe, settled and grounded. If you notice some discomfort after setting a boundary with someone or saying 'no' to an invite – maybe your heart is racing, or you've got goosebumps, or you're starting to sweat – take a moment to engage in something soothing to show your system that you are safe. You might want to make yourself a drink in your favourite mug, watch a comforting TV show or talk to a friend who 'gets it'. These can put the brakes on a nervous system that is about to spiral into anxiety or avoidance mode.

People-Pleasing

How it Looks

How it Feels

Easygoing

Fear of
abandonment

Difficulty
expressing
anger

Helpful

Flexible

Preoccupation
with what others
think of you

Considerate

Fear of being
disliked

Caring

Fear of conflict

Attentive

Polite

Learning to tolerate the discomfort of other people being disappointed or frustrated with us is one of the hardest things about deconstructing the people-pleasing pattern, but it's a powerful way to build resilience and reshape our system away from habitual fawning and people-pleasing behaviours.

Take a small step (and then another one)

Breaking the people-pleasing habit doesn't happen in a flash with one big action, but in little changes that add up over time. Your nervous system has become accustomed to you hyperfocusing on other people in order to feel safe and it will need time to adjust to you communicating your needs.

If you are new to pleasing yourself, you might want to start with something small: let a call go to voicemail, speak up about which restaurant you would prefer or schedule a meeting at a time that suits you. When you see how well most people respond to your boundaries, you will gain the confidence to keep practising and build up to something more challenging. You wouldn't go to the gym for the first time and start lifting the heaviest weights you could find. Ideally you would start with something that felt like a stretch, but that was also realistic. Any personal trainer will tell you that we want our muscles to feel a little bit sore after a good workout, but we don't want to push ourselves so hard that we get injured and set ourselves back. It's the same with learning to please ourselves: a small amount of discomfort is a sign that we're growing stronger and more resilient, but it's important that we find the right degree of challenge for our mind-body system. When it comes to changing deeply entrenched habits like people-pleasing, we need to be patient but persistent, and remember that small adjustments lead to transformational changes.

EXERCISE: CLEAR BOUNDARIES FOR PEOPLE-PLEASERS

Making a change in your life needs to start from somewhere, no matter how small. Think about one tiny way in which you can start to break your people-pleasing pattern today. This will be personal to you, but here are some ideas in case you're feeling stuck on where to start:

When a chatty colleague is affecting your productivity:

> *'Sorry, I'm swamped right now, but maybe we can catch up later?'*

When someone is giving you unwanted advice:

> *'I appreciate your concern, but this is my decision.'*

When someone speaks to you aggressively:

> *'I'm happy to have this conversation with you, but it's not okay for you to shout at me.'*

When we can reclaim our true wants and needs and learn that it is OK to disappoint people, or to be different, we can finally live in alignment with our true self and our values. We can reconnect with the lost parts of ourselves and build more genuine and fulfilling relationships with people. Authenticity is contagious. When we show people who we really are, we also give them permission to be real with us.

Hiding or contorting ourselves to please others may have felt like a route to safety but it ultimately leads to anxiety, loneliness, stress and a diminished sense of self. Putting down the people-pleasing shield and recovering our authentic self-expression is how we can feel more at ease in ourselves and spend more time hanging out in a state of regulation, where we feel calm, open, connected and safe. Teaching our nervous system that it's safe to state our boundaries or let ourselves be seen is a radical act of self-love and opens the door to a whole new world of opportunity and connection.

5.
PERFECTIONISM

If you are tempted to skip past this chapter because you don't consider yourself to be a perfectionist, I can relate. I was reluctant to identify with the label 'perfectionist' for a long time because I thought a perfectionist was someone who did everything *perfectly*. I often hear this from my clients too: '*I can't be a perfectionist, my room is always a mess!*'; '*I'm definitely not a perfectionist, my spelling and grammar is appalling!*' But perfectionism is not just about being obsessive and meticulous about small details, nor is it about striving to be our best.

> PERFECTIONISM IS ABOUT HOLDING OURSELVES TO UNNECESSARILY HIGH STANDARDS AND THEN CRITICISING OURSELVES WHEN WE FAIL TO PERFORM THE UNATTAINABLE.

Perfectionism can show up in our lives in myriad ways: our work; our appearance; how we appear on social media; how we parent; how we decorate our home; how we meditate; or even how conscientious or moral we appear to other people. There is a lot of secret striving involved in perfectionism but it doesn't make us feel happy and accomplished; it makes us feel as though we are always falling short, and it can feed an unhealthy obsession with how other people view us.

Perfectionism is a sign that we are disconnected from our true selves. As we will see, the paradox of perfectionism is that its pursuit does not lead to a full, rewarding and authentic life. Instead, it makes us highly self-critical, it dysregulates our nervous system and it impairs our ability to deeply connect with ourselves and the people around us. Part of reclaiming our authentic self involves rejecting the pressure to be flawless and accepting that we are enough, just as we are.

THE FEAR OF FAILURE

Much like people-pleasing, perfectionism is a coping mechanism to shield ourselves from pain and discomfort. We saw in the previous chapter that people-pleasing is the hope that if we can make everyone around us happy, we can avoid the discomfort of being disliked or abandoned. Perfectionism is similar, but it's the hope that if we can do things perfectly, we can avoid the discomfort of failure and criticism. As professor and author Brené Brown puts it, 'Perfectionism is a self-destructive and addictive belief system that fuels this primary thought: If I look perfect, live perfectly, work perfectly, and do everything perfectly, I can avoid or minimize the painful feelings of shame, judgement and blame.'

Perfectionism Can Show Up In Many Different Ways

Our work

How we parent

Our appearance

How we appear on social media

Our home

How moral we are

Our relationships

How conscientious we appear

Our mental health

CONTRARY TO THE NAME, MOST
PERFECTIONISTS ARE NOT DRIVEN BY
THE PURSUIT OF PERFECTION; THEY ARE
DRIVEN BY THE AVOIDANCE OF FAILURE.

An obsession with being flawless provides the semblance of a sense of control: If we never make a mistake, and we never give anyone a reason to criticise us, then we can stay away from uncomfortable feelings. But there is a major problem with this self-protective strategy: *perfection doesn't exist*. It is an unattainable goal. If we are constantly striving for perfection then we are setting ourselves up for failure because nothing in life is perfect and no one can do things perfectly. We cannot escape mistakes, failure, judgement and criticism – they are (whether we like it or not) unavoidable parts of life.

If you are a perfectionist, you'll likely often do more than is necessary and more than is healthy, perhaps working long hours, over-preparing, never delegating, or excessively exercising. You may often complain that you are unable to turn off your 'mental chatter' and lie awake at night compulsively thinking about how you need to work harder, do more and be better.

Perfectionism doesn't just lead to over-achieving though; it can also lead to procrastination and the avoidance of new experiences or opportunities. We avoid challenging tasks where we know we can't definitely fulfil them perfectly. The unconscious thinking behind our procrastinating is: '*If I don't try then I can't fail*'. In this sense, perfectionism keeps us in a small area of functioning that feels safe and secure, which is why many perfectionists wind up feeling very 'stuck' in their careers: you might never ask for a pay rise, put yourself up for a promotion or apply for a new job because you predict failure at every turn.

Perfectionism and the nervous system

Underneath perfectionism, there is a belief that we are inadequate, not good enough, or deficient in some way. When a perfectionist makes a mistake or fails (which is inevitable because perfection is an unattainable goal), they often find themselves in a dysregulated state and subject themselves to harsh self-criticism: *'You're an idiot'*; *'You messed everything up'*; *'You're useless'*. Rather than seeing a mistake as an opportunity to learn or grow, they see it as evidence that they are deeply flawed – it confirms their perceived inadequacy – and it can trigger deep feelings of shame. Therapist and nervous system specialist Deb Dana points out that from a nervous system perspective, perfectionism is an attempt to stay out of the autonomic shutdown state of collapse, where we experience feelings of shame or hopelessness. It's a safety-seeking behaviour. The unconscious thinking for perfectionists is *'I must never make a mistake, otherwise I will feel deeply inadequate and I will end up in shutdown mode, where I feel useless and ashamed.'*

An obsession with being perfect might keep perfectionists out of shutdown mode in the short term, but it does little to make them feel safe, settled and regulated. Most perfectionists spend a lot of time living in fight-or-flight mode – they are constantly 'on the go', running from failure and chasing perfection – which makes them very vulnerable to stress, anxiety and burnout.

Where perfectionism comes from

The good news is that perfectionism is not something we are born with. It is – like the fawn response – a learned behaviour. For some people, perfectionism is a result of having a perfectionistic parent when they were growing up. Perfectionism can first form with parents pushing their children to have perfect grades or perfect careers – all driven by the fear of future failure. This kind of pressure can set a child up to believe that if they don't achieve the highest standards, they aren't valued, and this can easily leak out into other corners of their life. The internalised belief is '*I need to be perfect to be loved*' or '*I need to be perfect to be seen.*' Sadly, many adults who grew up with perfectionistic parents are very disconnected from their true, authentic selves because they learned from a young age to put too much emphasis on things that look socially acceptable on the outside and not enough emphasis on the things that make them feel genuinely happy, fulfilled or regulated.

PARENTAL PRESSURE CAN SET A CHILD UP TO BELIEVE THAT IF THEY DON'T ACHIEVE THE HIGHEST STANDARDS, THEY AREN'T VALUED.

For others, perfectionism may be due to having a parent who was the opposite: out of control, emotionally explosive, unpredictable or abusive. Many children blame themselves for the bad things that happen to them and internalise the idea that they are deficient or not good enough, and perfectionism can become a way of warding off these painful feelings. It may seem odd that a child would blame themselves for bad things that happened to them, but there is actually a protective function to this kind of self-accusation. As a child, it is terrifying to believe that our parents are incapable of caring for us, and that the world is an unpredictable and dangerous place. Believing that bad things happened to us because we weren't good enough is somehow more bearable than the alternative – that the people we depended on were incapable of meeting our needs. Believing that the deficiency is ours at least gives us some explanation for the suffering we endured. It also gives us some hope and some semblance of control: maybe if we just do more, do better, we will be safe and loved.

Alternatively, some perfectionists were 'parentified' when they were growing up, which is when a child has to take care of the needs of their parent or their siblings. Parentification occurs when a child is put in a position where they have to 'grow up too soon' – they may have been their parents' emotional support system, been the mediator in family arguments, or been responsible for taking care of their siblings.

Parentification can happen for many reasons, such as divorce, financial hardship, the death of a caregiver/parent or sibling, substance abuse, mental or chronic illness, or disability of a parent or sibling. Growing up in an environment where the roles between a child and parent are reversed can establish a baseline of chaos and disorder – even when these roles happen as a result of necessity. The heart-breaking issue with parentification is that it sets the child up for failure because they are attempting to perform tasks that are beyond their capabilities. These children may *internalise* these failures, which can lead to self-esteem issues and feelings of

Parentification Typically Falls Into Two Categories

1 **Instrumental parentification:**

This is when a child or teen is given 'functional responsibilities' that aren't appropriate for their age, such as housework, cooking, taking care of siblings, caring for sick family members, taking themselves to the doctors, paying bills, and others 'adult' responsibilities.

2 **Emotional parentification:**

This is when a child or teen tries to fulfil the emotional needs of the parent. This might involve being the parent's emotional caretaker, counsellor or confidant. The parent might tell the child about their frustrations, fears or complain about their relationship.

inadequacy. It can also lead to perfectionistic issues with control. That is, if you grew up having to shoulder big responsibilities, you may have felt that everything was on you. So now, as an adult, you feel over-responsible for things and have a hard time letting go and trusting others to do things for themselves. You may feel you know what's best for other people and struggle to let others think for themselves. It should be noted that not all adults who were parentified or who experienced childhood trauma become perfectionists – some may forever find themselves in chaotic situations and environments because it feels familiar and therefore comfortable.

REFLECTING ON THE PAST ISN'T ABOUT BLAMING ANYONE; IT'S ABOUT UNDERSTANDING OURSELVES BETTER.

It might feel strange and unsettling to look back at your childhood in this way. If the topics of childhood trauma and parentification have brought up some vulnerable emotions or traumatic memories, it might be important to seek some regular therapy so that you have a supportive container to process what arises.

PERFECTIONISM AND RELATIONSHIPS

Whether you can determine where your perfectionism comes from, it's likely going to affect your relationships. Even though people with perfectionism present themselves in ways that they hope will gain approval and acceptance, it's a strategy that often backfires. Research has found that an unrealistic need for perfection can interfere with the way we connect with other people, which can lead to loneliness and a lack of belonging. There are a handful of reasons why perfectionism might lead to social disconnection. First, from the other person's perspective, it can be frustrating to be around a perfectionist who always complains that they are under stress and anxiety, but who refuses to surrender their exacting standards.

Second, it can be hard to relate to perfection. If someone is always promoting their talents and abilities in order to impress people, or if they are unwilling to share their flaws and vulnerabilities, they can come across as disingenuous. It can be challenging to form a meaningful bond with someone who presents themselves as flawless. There is a phenomenon in psychology called the Pratfall Effect, which states that making mistakes can make us *more* likeable. The theory was first suggested by psychologist Elliot Aronson in 1966, and the central idea is that being imperfect makes us less intimidating, more human and therefore more approachable. It's why we find it charming when someone can laugh at themselves and why we warm to celebrities who share unfiltered images of themselves.

Perfectionism can also make us lonely because it can interfere with the way we socialise. It has close ties with social anxiety, and many perfectionists will steer clear of parties, romantic dates, public speaking, exercise classes and other types of activities and relationships. This is because if you are a perfectionist, you might feel the need to wait until you embody your ideal version of who you think you are supposed to be. As a perfectionist, you might avoid signing up for a yoga class, for example, because you don't think you are flexible enough.

Or you may be hesitant to join a book club because you think you aren't smart enough. People often think that social anxiety is just about being shy, but it's actually the sense that if we don't do things perfectly, something embarrassing, deficient or flawed about us will become obvious to others.

If you struggle with social anxiety, you might hold yourself to strict rules and overly ambitious standards about how you socialise: '*I must always sound smart and funny*'; '*I must never appear anxious*'; '*There should never be awkward silences in conversations*'; '*My house must always be tidy when I'm entertaining*'. The pressure to socialise perfectly can drive us to avoid social situations altogether. After all, it's hard to find the motivation to socialise when we are putting pressure on ourselves to be perfect. Sadly, this is how perfectionism and social anxiety can shrink our lives and fuel loneliness.

Perfectionism can also interfere with our ability to connect with other people because it can manifest as being highly critical and judgemental of others. Perfectionists tend to approach the world in a very black-or-white way and often believe that there is a 'right' or 'wrong' way to do everything. If you're a perfectionist, this can make decisions about where to live, where to work or who to date incredibly anxiety-inducing because you see a risk of failure in every decision you make, and it can even make casual events like writing in a friend's birthday card or deciding what to wear in the morning unnecessarily stressful. But it can also impact the way you interact with other people. Many perfectionists project their own perfectionistic standards on to others and can walk around the world very critical of people who aren't doing things 'correctly'. This can lead to attempts

Signs Your Social Anxiety Is Making You Hypervigilant Around Other People

You feel as though everyone is judging you

You replay conversations in your mind

You constantly fear being ridiculed or embarrassed

You worry that people can see how anxious you are

You hyper-focus on others for signs of disapproval

You imagine people are talking about how awkward or boring you are

If You Experience Social Anxiety, Instead of Aiming for Perfection, Try Aiming for 'Good Enough'

Lower your bar for conversations and remind yourself that everyone has a responsibility to keep the conversation going, not just you.

Take the pressure off having a perfectly presented home every time you have people over, and remind yourself that everyone's homes get messy and imperfect.

Lower your standards for always making a good impression and remind yourself that social interactions are not a performance, they are simply about being with other people.

Go easy on yourself for appearing anxious and remind yourself that even if people can see that you feel anxious, it doesn't mean they will think badly of you.

to control situations and people: maybe you feel like your partner has to load the dishwasher a certain way; your neighbours don't use their bins correctly; your friends aren't taking care of their health properly, or people at work aren't sharing files in the exact right way.

> PERFECTIONISM CAN MANIFEST
> AS BEING HIGHLY CRITICAL AND
> JUDGEMENTAL OF OTHERS, WHICH
> CAN INTERFERE WITH OUR ABILITY TO
> CONNECT WITH OTHER PEOPLE.

Unfortunately, perfectionism is often at the expense of flexibility, openness and compassion towards other people, and it can really take its toll on our interpersonal relationships because people on the receiving end of perfectionism can feel controlled, judged and criticised. Perfectionistic controlling behaviour is usually an attempt to feel safe; to feel calm and regulated. For perfectionists, control plays an important part in their need for certainty and security, which is why it can be so hard to loosen their grip. We'll take a look at effective tools for tackling perfectionism after first looking at a closely related feeling: imposter syndrome.

IMPOSTER SYNDROME

Imposter syndrome is a psychological pattern in which an individual doubts their accomplishments or talents and has a persistent internalised fear of being exposed as a 'fraud'.

Imposter syndrome was first identified in 1978 by psychologists Pauline Rose Clance and Suzanne Imes. In their paper, they theorised that sufferers of imposter syndrome are convinced that their achievements are due to luck, timing or as a result of tricking others into thinking they are better than they believe themselves to be.

Imposter syndrome tends to get triggered when we are trying something new or when we are out of our comfort zone. In her book, *The Imposter Cure*, Dr Jessamy Hibberd points out that everyone feels anxious when they are out of their comfort zone, but people who suffer from imposter syndrome interpret this anxiety as meaning they are a fraud – they falsely believe that if they were good enough, they wouldn't feel anxious. The healthy reaction therefore would be to recognise that it's normal to feel anxious when we're outside of our comfort zone.

If you feel anxious when you start a new job, meet new people, travel to a new place or launch a new business venture, it doesn't mean you are not confident or capable enough, it means you are human. The effect of imposter syndrome – putting pressure on yourself to never feel out of your depth – is actually, in itself, a form of perfectionism.

Overcoming imposter syndrome involves recognising that anxiety is a valid and understandable response to uncertainty – it's our nervous system trying to keep us safe. It's not a sign that we can't cope. Remember, our mind-body system is always trying to keep us away from dangerous people, places and situations. When we do something new and unfamiliar, we may feel a spike in anxiety because our nervous system has been put on high-alert – it's scanning for threats in a bid to make

6 Common Experiences Associated With Imposter Syndrome

You doubt your accomplishments and live with an underlying fear that you will be exposed as a 'fraud' or a 'fake'.

You live with a voice in your head that is constantly telling you that you aren't good enough and that everyone is judging you.

You feel inadequate despite demonstrating competency.

You downplay or minimise your achievements because you believe your success is down to luck or good timing.

You constantly compare yourself to other people and always feel that you could have done more.

You are very sensitive to even constructive criticism and spend a lot of time overanalysing your performance.

sure this situation is safe. It's as though our nervous system is saying, '*Is this new situation dangerous? Are these new people safe? Is it OK to relax?*'

It's important to point out here that there are myriad systemic factors which create the sense of imposter syndrome for marginalised communities, causing feelings of inadequacy which are reflective of the flaws in the systems and structures that we operate in as society, based around gender, race, culture, inherited privilege and socioeconomic standing. This is beyond the scope of this book to delve into, but illustrates how internalised feelings of lack of worth or confidence can often be more about external systems around us.

PUTTING PRESSURE ON YOURSELF TO NEVER TO FEEL ANXIOUS IS A FORM OF PERFECTIONISM.

I remember feeling very anxious the evening before my first day as a new student on my psychotherapy training course. Instead of recognising that it was completely normal and understandable to feel anxious about embarking on something new, I made the mistake of misinterpreting my anxiety as a sign that I wasn't up to the task. I experienced a big wave of 'imposter feelings' and convinced myself that I wasn't good enough to do the training. I was scared that everyone was going to discover that I didn't belong or deserve to be there. The more I listened to these thoughts, the more my nervous system became dysregulated towards a hyperactive state of fight-or-flight. Rather than regulating my nervous system with rest and soothing activities,

I stayed up far too late frantically over-preparing, and woke up feeling anxious and exhausted, which did little for my confidence.

If I knew then what I know now about imposter syndrome and how my nervous system was working to protect me, I would have done things differently. I would recognise that everyone experiences anxiety when they are out of their comfort zone and I would speak to myself in a compassionate and reassuring way: *'I'm feeling anxious because I'm doing something new and my nervous system is working to protect me, it doesn't mean I'm not capable or good enough.'* This could have stopped any 'imposter thoughts' in their tracks and put the brakes on my urge to frantically over-function.

Instead of nervously busying myself with preparation the night before my first day, and further dysregulating my system, I could have chosen to engage in some regulating practices: have a bath; talk to someone about how I was feeling; or do a few breathing exercises or yoga poses before bed. It's the small actions that help soothe our nervous system and show our mind-body that we aren't under threat. These regulating practices won't always *eliminate* our anxiety, but they can help us keep it in check and *tolerate* the discomfort.

REMEMBER, RESILIENCE IS SOMETHING
WE CULTIVATE OVER TIME.

As soon as we take the pressure off ourselves to feel happy, confident and regulated all the time, we take a big step towards freeing ourselves from imposter syndrome. Reclaiming our authenticity means embracing all parts of us, especially the

3 Types of Imposter Feelings

FEELING LIKE A FAKE	ATTRIBUTING SUCCESS TO LUCK	DISCOUNTING SUCCESS
'I don't belong here'	'I just got lucky this time'	'It's not a big deal'
'It's only a matter of time before I get found out'	'I was in the right place at the right time'	'I just worked really hard'
'I fooled them'	'It was a fluke'	'I had a lot of help'

'imperfect' parts. The paradox is that when we accept that it's perfectly normal to feel anxious or stressed when we are out of our comfort zone, then we are more able to engage in regulating behaviours that will soothe our anxiety or stress.

As previously stated in earlier chapters, the more we deliberately show our nervous system that we are safe following a stressful experience, the more resilient our nervous system can become. Resilience doesn't mean never experiencing fear again; it means that when we do experience a dip into dysregulation, we can quickly bounce back to feeling calm and relaxed.

BE HONEST ABOUT YOUR PERFECTIONISM

Overcoming perfectionism isn't something that happens overnight – it's a process that requires plenty of self-compassion and often needs to be worked through with a therapist – but there are some steps you can take towards letting go of this destructive coping mechanism.

If we want to drop perfectionism, we need to be honest with ourselves about three things:

1. **What has my perfectionism cost me?** Ask yourself, what have I sacrificed or neglected because my perfectionism tells me I need to work harder, do more and prove myself? What opportunities or experiences have I missed because I'm afraid of failing? Has my perfectionism interfered with my relationships or my ability to connect with people?

2. **What do I get from my perfectionism?** Ask yourself, what am I getting versus what am I losing? Perfectionism will undoubtedly have some positives – it might give you a bump in your self-worth, a sense of control, or small dopamine hits when you are recognised as being perfect – but is this worth the costs: the chronic stress, anxiety, shame, envy, rumination, loneliness or exhaustion? Doing a cost/benefit analysis can help us see that while perfectionism might be understandable, it is ultimately self-harming.

3. **What are some of the benefits of letting go of perfectionism?** Ask yourself: Would I have more time for the things that I enjoy if I let go of perfectionism? Would I get along better with friends/partner/colleagues? Would I be less anxious? Would I enjoy my job more?

EXERCISE: GET TO KNOW YOUR PERFECTIONISM

Take some time to answer the three questions above, to try and get to the root of your perfectionism. The first step towards making a change is awareness, so gently probe into your perfectionist mindset to get a better picture of how it's affecting your life.

INTERNALISING YOUR SUCCESS

Many perfectionists – particularly those who struggle with imposter syndrome – can be very disconnected from their success.

One of the most effective ways to combat perfectionism is to therefore learn to accept and take pride in your achievements. Perfectionists tend to reject their success in a few different ways:

1. You might attribute your success to luck or good timing, believing you were just in the right place at the right time. You might say things like: *'I only got a promotion because my manager left'* or *'It was just a fluke'*.

2. Or you might discount your achievements altogether and, instead of attributing your success to hard work or intelligence, say things like: *'I just knew the right people'* or *'I only got a place at university because it was an unpopular course'*.

3. Or you might refuse to take credit if you received any kind of assistance, saying things like: *'It's no big deal, I had a lot of help'* or *'It was a team effort.'*

EXERCISE: ACCURATE ACHIEVEMENTS

Take a look at the three points above. Which of them resonates with you the most?

Admittedly, success can often be down to luck, good timing, privilege or support from other people, but these don't make up 100 per cent of your overall success. Hard work, curiosity, determination, perseverance and commitment also contribute to success. Take a moment to be honest about what you have accomplished – write down a few notes on what you have achieved this week, this month, this year. Doing this summary will give you a more accurate picture of your strengths so that you are no longer reliant on being recognised as being perfect in order to feel capable.

EMBRACING 'GOOD ENOUGH-NESS'

One of the other most effective tools for overcoming perfectionism is embracing 'good enough' – a concept derived from the work of a British psychoanalyst called Donald Winnicott in the 1950s. In his clinical practice, Winnicott saw a lot of parents who felt like they were failing their children, not because they were getting anything majorly wrong, but because they were putting a lot of pressure on themselves to be perfect parents. Winnicott developed his famous phrase 'the good enough parent' to help his clients escape damaging perfectionistic standards. Winnicott insisted that children don't need 'ideal' parents, who are tirelessly responsive and selfless; they just need OK, well-intentioned, 'good enough' parents. His theory wasn't about telling people to settle for poor parenting; it was about helping them recognise that perfectionism is damaging and counterproductive.

EXERCISE: CHOOSE TO DO SOMETHING IMPERFECTLY

The concept of 'good enough' is something that is often learned in therapy and it can be applied to all aspects of life. You can be a good enough partner, friend, employee, sister, cook, writer or runner. When I have a client who struggles with perfectionism, I like to invite them to try out a 'behavioural experiment' inspired by Winnicott's concept, in which they intentionally do things imperfectly.

Instead of aiming for 100 per cent, aim for 80 per cent and see what happens. Here are some ways you might do this:

- Leave a typo on a document for a client

- Leave the house without your usual full face of make-up

- Invite friends rounds for a takeaway instead of cooking something elaborate

- Don't overtidy your home before having friends or family over

- Stop exercising earlier than you'd planned, for example, go for a 20-minute run instead of 30 minutes.

People are often amazed to see that nothing disastrous happens when they scale back. In fact, they usually realise that nobody even noticed or cared that they didn't give 100 per cent, and they relish all the extra time they have to do something more valuable. People also often find that when they stop pulling out all the stops in their career, they are actually more productive. When you spend three hours on something instead of five, you open yourself up to getting more work done.

Don't be discouraged if you feel anxious the first time you do something imperfectly – your nervous system has become accustomed to you striving for perfection at all costs and your body will be on the lookout for judgement or criticism when you first start experimenting with imperfection. When this happens, try not to let the anxiety pull you back into a place of exacting standards. Instead, pause for a moment and ask yourself, how can I calm myself and tolerate this discomfort?

DEVELOPING A GROWTH MINDSET

If we want to crawl out from perfectionistic standards, we need to learn to take criticism, mistakes and failure in our stride. Perfectionists often see failure as a dead-end. In psychology this is called having a 'fixed mindset' – it's the belief that talent and intelligence are fixed, so when we fail or make a mistake it's as evidence that we are inadequate. It's much healthier to have a 'growth mindset' – when we see our flaws and mistakes as opportunities for growth. When we have a growth mindset, we accept that setbacks are part of the learning process. The truth is, learning to fail is a skill like any other. It takes practice but once you know how to do it, you can recognise the hidden benefits of failure and change your mindset from one of fear to one of adventure.

* * *

Growth Mindset vs Fixed Mindset

GROWTH MINDSET	FIXED MINDSET
Believes that intelligence and talent can be developed over time	Believes that intelligence and talent are fixed
Embraces flaws and mistakes as opportunities for growth	Hides flaws and mistakes and feels ashamed about 'failures'
Embraces challenges and is willing to risk possible failure	Avoids challenges to prevent the possibility of failure
Views feedback as an opportunity to grow and learn	Views feedback as a personal attack
Finds inspiration in other people's success	Feels threatened by other people's success

EXERCISE: **FIND YOUR MANTRA**

Whenever you feel a perfectionism attack coming on, it can be useful to have a mantra or two to say out loud or in your head. Next time you notice that you are putting too much pressure on yourself or that you are setting yourself unrealistically high standards, these mantras can help you gain perspective, remain focused and stay regulated.

- *Nothing in life is perfect*

- *I do not have to be perfect to be safe or loved*

- *I have the right to make mistakes*

- *Progress, not perfection, is what matters*

- *Every mistake is an opportunity to practice being kind to myself*

- *Being imperfect doesn't mean I'm a fraud.*

- *Not everything deserves 100 per cent*

- *Good enough is good enough*

- *It doesn't have to be perfect to be powerful*

6.
BUSYNESS

We don't often talk about it, but many of us assume that being busy means we are living our 'best lives'. We are a society *obsessed* with getting things done. From 'brain power'-boosting supplements to time management apps, the ability to be productive at all times can feel like evidence that we are on the road to success. If we are not careful, this obsession with achieving things can take over our lives and leave us stranded in states of 'productivity anxiety', where we feel anxious and self-critical about not getting enough done.

Far too many of us have bought into the faulty belief that our self-worth is tied to our output, and that we need to be as productive as possible in order to be successful. In many ways, we wear our busyness as a badge of honour. Our jam-packed schedules have become status symbols, and we can find ourselves in a pit of shame if we think we're not achieving enough. Admittedly, there is nothing wrong with being busy and productive – it can sometimes boost our self-esteem and release feel-good endorphins – but when we are convinced that every minute of 'empty time' in our lives must be pointed towards achievement or self-improvement, we can start filling our days with activities that detach us from our true self.

MANY OF US ARE SO BUSY BEING BUSY THAT WE DON'T TAKE THE TIME TO REFLECT ON WHAT ACTUALLY MAKES US HAPPY, AND WE BARELY NOTICE THAT WE'RE LIVING IN AN ALMOST PERMANENT STATE OF FIGHT-OR-FLIGHT, AFRAID TO TAKE OUR FOOT OFF THE GAS.

SOME COMMON SIGNS OF PRODUCTIVITY ANXIETY:

- The first thing you think about when you wake up is how much is on your to-do list

- The last thing you think about before you go to sleep is that you didn't tick enough items off your to-do list

- You feel guilty or 'lazy' for taking time off to rest, even if you are ill

- You believe that the more you do, the happier you will be

- You feel 'tired and wired' because you struggle to switch off and relax if you think you haven't achieved enough

- You view the basics like sleep and nutrition as fuel so you can get more done (instead of as ways to create more health and pleasure in your body)

I used to suffer from toxic busyness and productivity anxiety. I spent a lot of time living in overdrive. I was so focused on optimising my time that I was never really resting. I would eat my lunch while staring at a spreadsheet and I would watch TV while answering emails on my phone. I was so programmed to make every moment 'count' that even when I went for a walk, I would try to optimise the time by returning a phone call or listening to an educational podcast. I thought my obsession with productivity was making me happy, but it was making me feel on-edge and lacking. My over-familiarity with fight-or-flight meant that even when I tried to slow down, I would feel bored or uneasy, and find myself gravitating towards hyper-activity again. I was addicted to my own adrenaline (the hormone released when our body shifts into fight-or-flight).

It's easy to fall into the trap of believing that the busier we are, the more satisfied and fulfilled we will be. There is a lot of societal pressure to be constantly productive, but chronic stress and trauma can all cause us to live a frantic, hurried life. If we want to reclaim our time, our energy and our life, we need to take a step back and recognise that our value and worth as a person does not depend on being busy all of the time.

HIGH-FUNCTIONING ANXIETY

An obsession with being busy is also part of the experience of 'high-functioning anxiety'. High-functioning anxiety isn't an official diagnosis; it's a term that is used to describe someone who lives with persistent anxiety but functions relatively well in different areas of their life. The way high-functioning anxiety manifests internally is very different to how it is expressed externally, so those who struggle with it are able to conceal it well. Internally, there can be racing thoughts, intense fears, increased heart rate and even insomnia. Yet externally, a person may seem to be excelling in life and appear the height of professionalism: calm; composed; and immaculately put together.

A fitting way to describe someone with high-functioning anxiety is like a swan gliding across a river. The animal appears serene and graceful on the outside, but just beneath the surface, it's furiously kicking its legs to stay moving. Many people with high-functioning anxiety spend a lot of time in fight-or-flight mode, frantically overworking and trying to 'prove' themselves, but then 'crashing' at the end of the day or week, and finding themselves in a shutdown state of collapse, where they feel withdrawn, lethargic and emotionally flat. This nervous system rollercoaster ride can drive many people to self-regulate with alcohol or drugs, which only perpetuates the problem. Further on in the chapter, we'll take a look at healthier ways to cope, if high-functioning anxiety resonates with you.

Job entanglement

One reason it can be difficult to unsubscribe from chronic busyness and live a more balanced life is to do with how closely we identify with our job. For many of us, our careers are about much more than how we pay the bills, and doing work that we love is an important part of our identity and how we spend our time – it certainly is for me. But when we define ourselves *exclusively* by our job, we can slide into the dangerous territory

High-Functioning Anxiety

HOW IT CAN LOOK		HOW IT CAN FEEL
Hardworking		Fear of failure
Full of energy		Difficulty switching off
Organised		Need for control
Detail-oriented		Overthinking
'Yes' person		Fear of saying 'no'
Perfectionist		Fear of failure and criticism

of 'enmeshment' and become disconnected from our wholeness and who we are outside of our work.

In a *Harvard Business Review* article titled 'What Happens When Your Career Becomes Your Whole Identity?', Dr Janna Koretz explains that when people identify too closely with their role at work, they can become 'enmeshed' with their job, which makes them vulnerable to anxiety, burnout and painful identity issues. Psychotherapists normally use the term 'enmeshment' in the context of families or romantic relationships to describe a situation where the boundaries between people are blurred, and independent identities are lost. When we experience enmeshment with our job, however, it is the line between our work and our personal life that is blurred.

People who are enmeshed in their jobs allow work to eat up all their time and identity and have very little space for downtime or hobbies. They might send emails at all hours or forget to take all of their allocated holiday days. Or they might bring up their job within minutes of talking to someone or find it hard to connect with people who aren't part of their working life. It's OK to have a strong sense of connection to your job; it can yield some positive results. Caring deeply about your work can increase motivation and dedication, and allow you to experience a sense of meaning and purpose, but when you are so enmeshed in your job that it *defines* you, it can have a negative effect on your mental health and sense of individuality.

People who are overly attached to their work often get trapped in a self-perpetuating cycle of stress, where they are afraid that if they stop, they will experience some discomfort – perhaps a sense of emptiness, anxiety or boredom – so they

5 Common Faulty Beliefs That Can Lead to Burnout

'Exhaustion is the price of success'

'I'm more productive when I'm living in overdrive'

'I love my job so I won't burn out'

'Ambitious people are always tired'

'If I slow down, I'll lose momentum and fail'

keep pushing through the busyness and convince themselves that they will rest and play when they are 'done': *'I'll make more time to relax as soon as I get promoted'*; *'I'll see more of my friends and family when things slow down at work'*; or *'I can't stop now, there's too much to do'*. The problem with this approach is that they work and work, and climb and climb, until they become accustomed to a constant state of exhaustion – or worse, they hit complete burnout. Even for those who don't burn out, work enmeshment can still be problematic. When someone's work defines their value, and they haven't developed a sense of identity outside of their job, they can experience depression and a deep sense of loss when they retire, or when forced to take time off due to stress; or even when they go on holiday.

IF WE WANT TO RECLAIM OUR TIME, OUR ENERGY AND OUR LIFE, WE NEED TO TAKE A STEP BACK AND RECOGNISE THAT OUR VALUE AND WORTH AS A PERSON DOES NOT DEPEND ON BEING BUSY ALL OF THE TIME.

Detaching from work

If you want to untangle yourself from your job and reconnect with who you are outside of your work, you may need to intentionally create some space between your work life and your personal life. This may sound simple, but when our nervous system is accustomed to constant 'grind', work-life balance can be surprisingly difficult to achieve. Detaching from work begins with being honest with yourself about how much of your life is

6 Subtle Signs of Burnout That Mean You Need to Prioritise Rest

You can't make any decisions. Even something as simple as what to get for lunch feels overwhelming

You find it hard to get excited about anything

You feel insecure about things that you used to feel confident about

You feel extra sensitive and take everything personally

You are snappy and impatient with others

You have fallen back into unhealthy patterns

filled by work, then asking yourself what kind of boundaries you could set about separating from work.

Here are some examples of how you can set boundaries to help you detach from work:

Create friction between you and your work. If you struggle to switch off from work in the evenings and weekends, you might need to create some deliberate barriers between you and your work. Try deleting work-related apps from your phone, either permanently or just for the time you want to detach, and if you want to use your laptop when you're not working, use a different browser that doesn't have all your work-related bookmarks.

Have a transitional ritual. Switching off from work is even harder when our dining table is our office. If you work from home, do something concrete at the end of the day to mark the shift out of work time: go on a short walk; change your clothes; put your laptop out of sight. You can also signal to your body that it's time to switch off from work by using sensory cues, like different lighting, music, drinks or scents.

Remember that not everything is urgent. One of the reasons we get sucked back into work during our downtime is because we falsely believe that everything is pressing and high-priority – a hallmark of the fight-or-flight response. Try to identify what is urgent and what can wait for tomorrow. If your job involves monitoring an inbox, remember that if an email doesn't require your immediate attention but you still feel you need to respond, it's OK to reply with, *'I have seen your email and I will respond* *with an answer tomorrow*' or set an out-of-office letting people know a realistic time when you'll get back to them.

Limit the way you talk about your job with others. A healthy amount of venting can be helpful, but try not to dwell on issues. Ruminating can make us feel more stressed and keep our nervous systems in a revved-up state. Try to complain with perspective, which means recognising that while your work is important, it's not the only thing you have.

Another way to separate yourself from an unhealthy attachment to work is to explore your core values. Ask yourself, what is important to me? What do I value? What do I stand for? What do I want my life to be about?

See if you can let these priorities guide you towards a life outside of your job. Identifying what matters to you – whether that's honesty, friendship, creativity, social justice, environmentalism, kindness (there's an endless list to choose from) – helps you create the future you want. If you realise that your obsession with work has pulled you away from your core values, try not to shame or criticise yourself, as this will only make you feel worse. Instead, try to see this as an exciting opportunity to reconnect with who you are at your core and to build a life that aligns with your true goals and desires. When we are stressed and busy, it's easy to lose sight of who we are or why we do what we do, but it's never too late to reel ourselves back to a place where our values drive our decisions.

Ask Yourself...

What is important to me?

What do I stand for?

What do I value?

What do I want my life to be about?

WHY IT'S HARD TO SLOW DOWN

Many of us struggle to slow down and do less simply because we find it hard to sit with ourselves in our silence. In fact, we may do anything to avoid stillness, but why do we find this state of quiet so difficult to tolerate? Because when we remove all of the busyness, noise and distractions, we make space for uneasy thoughts and feelings to arise. It's why many people avoid meditating or feel the need to listen to music or a podcast while walking somewhere. We are so addicted to 'doing' that simply 'being', and allowing our emotions to come to the surface, can feel excruciating.

You may convince yourself that your 'go-go-go' approach to life is keeping you buoyant above uncomfortable feelings, depressive moods, or anxious thoughts. You may even depend on stimulating substances to keep your busyness afloat, but the truth is, no matter how much you stay busy and keep moving, you can't ever escape difficult thoughts and feelings. They will just come back, over and over again, getting louder and louder, often in the form of physical symptoms, until we finally give them the attention they need.

Your urgency and busyness make sense – it's your body's way of protecting you from the uncomfortable feelings that arise when we are undistracted. But we shouldn't be afraid to stop and listen to our internal world. When you pay attention to your inner world, you might discover some important truths – perhaps that you need to set some boundaries, do some more grieving, or heal some emotional wounds. Your inner compass might tell you that you need to leave your job, end a relationship, or make some important lifestyle changes.

UNEASY THOUGHTS AND FEELINGS AREN'T ENEMIES TO AVOID, THEY ARE FRIENDS WITH VALUABLE INFORMATION.

One of the reasons we run from our feelings is that we're afraid that if we stop and listen, we will need to make some difficult or uncomfortable changes. But we don't need to start wielding a wrecking ball. Slowing down and listening to our needs – and then honouring them – can be a gentle process, but it's also a powerful way to heal and grow; and an essential step on the path to reclaiming our happiness.

Gently start listening

One of the best ways to slow down and reconnect with our true self is to make stillness part of our daily lives. The concept of stillness is simple but for many people, including myself, it's not so easy to put into practice. Even though I intellectually understand that quiet reflection, alone time and meditation are powerful ways to quiet the body and mind in order to feel less anxious or overwhelmed, I still sometimes struggle to do it. I tell myself that I don't have the time to 'do nothing' or that if I slow down, I'll lose momentum and 'drop a ball'. Over the years, I resisted stillness so much by finding all kinds of reasons to justify living in overdrive: '*The adrenaline helps me reach my goals*'; '*I'm more productive when I'm stressed*'; '*Anxiety actually propels me forward*' (classic arguments from a 'busy-aholic'!). The truth is, when I spoke to myself like this, I was fearful of the discomfort I felt if I slowed down. My nervous system was

If You Struggle to Find Moments of Stillness In Your Day, Here are a Few Small Things You Can Do to Get Started

1. Next time you are standing in a queue for something, try to resist the urge to look at your phone, and instead, just be present with your thoughts.

2. When you are having your morning tea or coffee, take five minutes to sit quietly without any distractions and notice how you feel in your body.

3. Use your senses to help ground you – light a candle and spend a little time watching its flame, or apply a scented moisturiser to your body and spend a few moments smelling its aroma.

4. Sit in the sunshine and focus on the feeling of warmth on your face.

so accustomed to being in a permanent state of fight-or-flight that stillness actually felt *dangerous*.

If we want to walk away from toxic busyness and reclaim inner calm, we need to create capacity in our nervous system for stillness. This means *gently* building a tolerance for being present with our thoughts and feelings. As with any new habit, we need to start small.

CREATING CAPACITY IN OUR NERVOUS SYSTEM FOR STILLNESS WILL HELP US TO WALK AWAY FROM TOXIC BUSYNESS AND RECLAIM INNER CALM.

As you build more capacity for stillness in your life, your practices will become stronger, longer, and more habitual. Creating tiny pockets of stillness in your day-to-day life might seem pointless at first, but I can assure you, they will help you make the transition from chronic stress to inner balance.

I will say it again, because it is important: If we want to let go of busyness and productivity anxiety as a lifestyle, and reconnect with our inner wisdom, we need to introduce stillness into our lives *slowly*. Suddenly attempting 30 minutes of meditation or forcing ourselves to do a half-hour breathwork session can feel overwhelming to a nervous system that is regularly dysregulated towards fight-or-flight. Overloading your system like this can actually lead to *more* dysregulation: more anxiety, more shame, more avoidance. When we have lived chronically in states of busyness as a form of self-protection, our nervous system hasn't experienced enough 'proof' that the present moment is safe; and we need to gently allow our nervous system to feel safe in the 'here and now'. When it comes to reshaping our nervous system, the 'go hard or go home' mentality simply doesn't work. In order to create meaningful, lasting change, we need to do as Deb Dana suggests, and 'stretch, not stress' our system.

As you build your tolerance for being present with your thoughts and feelings, you will start to become more curious about your internal world, and even start to feel grateful for the information you are receiving. Rather than viewing your uneasy feelings as irritants to squash, you will start to see them as helpful clues about what you need to do or change. The coronavirus pandemic forced many of us to hit the pause button and pay attention to some thoughts and feelings we had been inadvertently running from. During the lockdowns, many of my clients found that getting off the hamster wheel, and living a slower-paced life, allowed them to become conscious of what aspects of their life were no longer serving them, and reconnect with parts of themselves they had severed. The bottom line is this: there are certain elements of ourselves and our lives that we can't reclaim when we are constantly on the go. It's fine to work hard and have periods of busyness, but if we never step off the treadmill, we're just running further and further away from who we really are at our core. As Eckhart Tolle says, 'When you lose touch with inner stillness, you lose touch with yourself.'

Reflecting on our internal world in a way that is curious and supportive doesn't just allow us to reclaim our truth and rebalance our nervous system, it also improves our relationships with others. People often find that when they learn to listen

to themselves with compassionate curiosity, rather than judgement, they learn to be more patient and accepting towards other
people too. When we look at others through a lens of compassionate curiosity, we are able to see someone who is struggling
and not make a judgement about who they are as a person. We
all want to feel safe and be loved, and we all have a nervous
system that can get stuck in survival mode.

SELF-CARE ANXIETY

When we start putting our boundaries in place, and experiencing the benefits of taking care of ourselves, it can also lead
to obsessive behaviours. Ironically, the pressure to practise
'self-care' can fuel toxic busyness and productivity anxiety. The
principles of hustle culture – go faster, get better, work harder
– have unfortunately bled into the ways in which 'self-care' is
marketed. Taking better care of yourself – exercising more,
resting more, eating better – is a crucial part of improving your
mental health and reclaiming your life. But when self-care
rituals and therapies become yet more items to 'tick off' your
to-do list, or they put a strain on your finances, they could be
doing more harm than good. Mindlessly rushing through yoga
sequences or overspending on every new wellness supplement
will do little to soothe a wigged-out nervous system. Constantly
pursuing self-care practices in the hope that all of our issues
will be resolved is dangerous because it distances us from our
true self and it pushes us into a space of believing that we are
'broken' and need 'fixing'.

Self-care doesn't have to be expensive and convoluted, and it certainly shouldn't be a source of stress or shame. Can you pause right now and ask yourself if your 'self-care' practices are *actually* contributing to your well-being?

REAL SELF-CARE IS ABOUT TUNING INTO YOURSELF AND LISTENING TO WHAT YOU REALLY NEED IN THE MOMENT.

Is that spin class truly what you need today, or is your nervous system craving something more soothing? Is buying the latest piece of wearable tech really what you need in order to feel healthy, or would you benefit more from putting that money towards a holiday? Is a night on the sofa with Netflix really what your body is calling for, or would you feel more regulated if you spoke to a friend about how you are feeling? Using cues from our nervous system – noticing what state our body is in – to guide our self-care choices is how we can embrace practices that are truly nourishing, like rest, nature, movement, connection and self-acceptance, rather than cramming our schedule full of activities that actually undermine our wellness.

THE SEVEN TYPES OF REST

One of the most underrated forms of self-care and a necessary antidote to a frantic state of busyness is rest. When we live in a frantic state of busyness, or we find it difficult to detach ourselves from our work, prioritising rest is very important.

Contrary to popular belief, rest isn't just about sleeping or relaxing at the weekend, it's about choosing the *right kind* of restorative activities that our whole mind-body system require. In her book, *Sacred Rest: Recover Your Life, Renew Your Energy, Restore Your Sanity*, Dr Saundra Dalton-Smith presents the idea that we all need seven different types of rest to feel fully rested and fully ourselves. According to Dalton-Smith, we must identify the type of rest we need and schedule it into our day:

1. **Physical rest:** This is the type of rest that relieves your body of physical stress, such as muscle tension, headaches, and a lack of sleep. Physical rest can be 'passive' (like sleeping or napping) or 'active' (like stretching, yoga, or warm baths).

2. **Social rest:** This type of rest isn't about taking a break from socialising; it's about spending time with people who don't need anything from you, where you just enjoy each other's company. It means limiting your exposure to toxic people, who drain your energy, and spending time with people you can relax with and be your true self.

3. **Mental rest:** This type of rest involves giving your brain a break from the 'mental chatter' or from thinking or focusing too hard. Meditation, time away from technology, or paying attention to the sensations in your body can quiet the mental noise and allow you to focus on what's really important.

4. **Emotional rest**: This type of rest involves authentically expressing and processing your emotions and eliminating people-pleasing behaviours. We experience emotional fatigue when we bottle up our feelings or put other people's needs ahead of our own.

5. **Creative rest:** Creative rest involves exposing yourself to inspiring environments without feeling the need to produce a creation. Creative rest can involve doing anything that helps you feel inspired, such as nature, an art gallery, or a creative hobby.

6. **Spiritual rest:** This type of rest involves connecting with something larger than yourself. It might mean practising your religion or engaging with something that gives you a sense of purpose, whether through community or though work where you feel like what you do matters.

7. **Sensory rest:** Sensory rest is the opportunity to give your senses a break (e.g. from technology, bright lights and loud noises). People who need sensory rest may find that they feel good at the beginning of the day, but can't understand why at the end of the day they are so agitated or irritable.

It was a revelation for me to realise that resting isn't just about getting eight hours sleep or having a quiet night in front of the TV, and that, in order to feel truly replenished, I needed to schedule the correct kind of restorative activities into my day. Once I made this mindset shift, I was able to regulate my nervous system and recharge my energy a lot more effectively. For example, these days, if I've had a day of back-to-back Zoom calls, I know that I will need some sensory rest in the evenings. For me, that means that taking a bath or reading a book is going to be much more restorative than sitting in front of the TV. Or if I've had a restless night's sleep because my mind has been racing, I will plan some activities that give my brain a break – perhaps 10 minutes of meditation before work or a 'mindful commute', where I focus on being present to my surroundings and the sensations in my body, rather than scrolling on Instagram. I don't always make the perfect choices when it comes to rest, but what I love about Dr Saundra Dalton-Smith's concept is that it encourages us to become mindful of how the energy we are using throughout the day is impacting our whole mind-body system, rather than simply declaring ourselves 'tired' and in need of sleep.

Gentle Reminders About Busyness

Having an identity outside of your work is a protective factor against burnout

You have the right to slow down and not always be productive

We often overwork because it feels easier to 'do' than to feel

Rest is required for growth

Life is for living, not just for achieving

Pressing pause allows us to listen to our inner wisdom

Rest isn't just about sleeping – we need to incorporate the *right type* of rest into our day

Slow and steady is more sustainable than busy and exhausted

EXERCISE: **REST THAT WORKS FOR YOU**

When we feel overwhelmed, it can be hard to choose what type of rest we need. To prepare for when you feel like this, use the different types of rest as a framework to make your own personalised list for different occasions.

Here are some examples to get you started:

- When I need creative rest, I will … walk in nature/visit an art gallery

- When I need sensory rest, I will … have a candlelit bath, turn off my phone for the evening

- When I need physical rest, I will … have a massage/attend a yoga class/go to bed early

- When I need mental rest, I will … journal before going to sleep/spend some time alone

7.
NUMBING

We all numb our feelings from time to time. If I'm completely honest, I used to do it frequently. Whenever a difficult feeling bubbled up, I would reach for Netflix, chocolate, online shopping, or a glass of wine – anything that would dial down my feelings of sadness, anger, disappointment, shame, or whatever other emotion I didn't want to feel. I think everyone falls somewhere on the 'numbing as a coping strategy' continuum. Some people only numb when they are feeling particularly overwhelmed or vulnerable. For others, numbing is compulsive and chronic, which is what we call addiction. Regardless of where we fall on the continuum, if we want to reclaim our true selves, we need to start being mindful about how much we are taking the edge off our painful feelings and learn to increase our capacity for sitting with discomfort. It's a common misconception that feeling numb means we have no emotions. The opposite is actually true.

Numbing is an attempt – albeit a misguided one – to feel safe. When we use alcohol, drugs, food, sex, gaming, scrolling, or anything else to dampen our feelings, we are seeking a way to soothe our nervous system. If we feel anxious, we might reach for the booze as a way to decompress, or if we feel sad, we might try to comfort ourselves by binge-watching a TV series. Distraction in moderation is OK – it can sometimes prevent us from becoming overwhelmed – but when we respond to our emotional pain by anesthetising ourselves, we are perpetuating our pain.

FEELING NUMB ISN'T ABOUT THE
ABSENCE OF EMOTIONS;
IT'S A RESPONSE TO EMOTIONS.

Emotionally detaching can feel good in the short term but there are a few major flaws in the strategy of numbing. First, numbing our emotions doesn't make them disappear. All we are doing when we numb our pain is temporarily muting it. In fact, numbing our emotions is counterproductive because when we avoid our feelings, they tend to come back stronger. If you are pushing down your shame, sadness or loneliness, or any other difficult emotion, you will notice it coming back over and over again, often in a much worse way. It's why, in part, we might feel particularly miserable when we are hungover or why we might be plagued by feelings of shame after we've over-indulged on sugar. Our dark feelings will come to the fore as soon as our 'drug' of choice fails.

Here is an analogy I find helpful: Imagine you are standing in a swimming pool and holding a beach ball under the water. The beach ball represents a feeling you are trying to get rid of. As long as you can hold the ball underwater, the surface of the water appears calm and smooth. In the short term this might not feel difficult and can even feel good, but your actions in the pool are limited – you are unable to move around freely and you can't hold the ball underwater forever. When you inevitably let go, the ball bursts up to the surface, creating a big splash. All of your feelings come to the surface and it can feel overwhelming and messy. This can lead to a vicious cycle as you try to frantically shove the ball underwater again. Sadly, this is how many people get trapped in a cycle of numbing that leads to addiction: the feelings they were trying to banish keep popping back up, in more painful ways, so they turn to stronger numbing agents, or they numb-out more frequently in order to push away their painful feelings. It's why trauma and addiction expert Dr Gabor Maté has the compassionate mantra, 'Not why the addiction, but why the pain'. Numbing is always about escaping something.

IN REDISCOVERING DIFFICULT FEELINGS
LIKE ANGER, SHAME OR SADNESS,
WE ALSO REDISCOVER JOY, PLEASURE
AND EXCITEMENT.

Another problem with numbing our emotions is to do with the fact that when we dull the difficult emotions, we unintentionally dull the pleasurable ones too. As Brené Brown says in *Dare to Lead*, 'We cannot selectively numb emotion. If we numb the dark, we numb the light. If we take the edge off pain and discomfort, we are, by default, taking the edge off joy, love, belonging and the other emotions that give meaning to our lives.'

In other words, we can't just say: *'I'm going to eat this packet of biscuits and mindlessly scroll on social media for a few hours to numb my sadness and loneliness, but I'm still going to fully experience joy and happiness!'* When we push one feeling under the surface, we push them all under the surface. In therapy, it can be a significant turning point for people when they come to the emotional insight that they have been inadvertently numbing their positive emotions. It may seem counterintuitive, but when we rediscover difficult feelings like anger, shame, or sadness, we also rediscover joy, pleasure and excitement. When we stop habitually numbing, we reclaim our vitality and our wholeness.

GLIMMERS VS NUMBING

There is nothing wrong with wanting to comfort ourselves when we are having a rough day. And sometimes that might mean we reach for the chocolate cake or the Nintendo Switch – those things aren't inherently bad. We just need to be careful that the ways we are choosing to soothe ourselves aren't making us feel much worse. The question is: where is the line between self-soothing and numbing? I get asked this question a lot and I believe the answer lies, to a large extent, with our nervous system. Before we dive in, let's start by briefly revisiting the three states of the nervous system we covered in Part 1:

Safe-and-social (the 'ventral vagal' state)

This is the state we are in when we feel happy, relaxed and grounded. When we are in the safe-and-social state our nervous system is regulated: we feel positive, compassionate and able to connect with other people. It's the 'sweet zone' where we feel calm, present, creative and able to focus.

Fight-or-flight (the 'sympathetic' state)

This is the state we are in when we feel anxious, stressed or angry. We move into this state when our nervous system detects a threat (real or perceived). When we are in fight-or-flight mode we might be consumed by worried thoughts, feel on-edge or irritable. We might find it impossible to focus or sit still and struggle to switch off and relax. When we are in fight-or-flight mode our nervous system is dysregulated: we lose our sense of being safe.

Shutdown (the 'dorsal vagal' state)

This is the state we are in when we feel depressed, hopeless or have no energy to do even the simplest thing. We might feel spaced-out, disconnected, and have no desire to connect with people. Just like fight-or-flight mode, shutdown mode is a dysregulated state we go into when we feel threatened. But rather than feeling 'switched on', like we do in fight-or-flight mode, we feel 'switched off' – like we've collapsed or disappeared.

Most of the time, whether we are conscious of it or not, we are on a mission to be in the safe-and-social state; the nervous system 'sweet zone'. We want our nervous system to be regulated; the goal is to feel safe. As we saw in Chapter 3, the best way to regulate and rebalance our nervous system after we have dropped into fight-or-flight or shutdown mode is to use our glimmers. (See page 50 if you need a reminder on these.) They are the practices that regulate our nervous system, moving our body into a feeling of safety and connection. Everyone has different glimmers – yours might be yoga, nature, a heart-to-heart with your best friend, deep breathing exercises or your favourite movie. So, how do we know that when we are using our glimmers, we are not subconsciously numbing ourselves from uncomfortable feelings?

When we are numbing, like using our glimmers, we are seeking a sense of safety. The unconscious thinking is *'I don't like this feeling of anger/anxiety/loneliness/<insert uncomfortable emotion>, so I'm going to make myself feel better by drinking this beer/eating this ice cream/playing this video game/<insert your go-to numbing device>'*. Whether we are aware of it or not, we are trying to regulate our nervous system by turning to certain behaviours or substances that take the edge off our uncomfortable feelings. But, when we are numbing, we are only making things worse. Rather than signalling to our body that we are safe, we are sending a message that there is something dangerous we need to *hide* from. When we are numbing, we are trying to do two related things: escape feelings of threat; and pursue feelings of safety. We are simply on a quest to feel good. This reframe can be very helpful for those of us who shame ourselves for compulsively numbing because it can help us see the process of numbing not as 'bad', but as understandable in terms of attempts to feel better.

Numbing is an ineffective game-plan for becoming regulated. The substitution of healthy glimmers with a strategy of squashing our feelings down will always fail because our numbing behaviours don't infuse our nervous system with experiences of safety; they further dysregulate our nervous system. They reinforce a sense of threat and take us away from the present moment. Bingeing on wine and pizza might help you stuff down your feelings of loneliness, or temporarily silence your self-critical thoughts, but it's not guiding your nervous system towards the safe-and-social state, where you feel present, calm and connected. It's pushing your nervous system into either shutdown mode, where you feel disconnected, withdrawn or foggy, or into fight-or-flight mode, where you feel on edge, irritable or chaotic. Many people find this difficult to accept at first (myself included!) because numbing feels effective in the short term – it can provide temporary relief or pleasure – but the truth is, it does little to promote feelings of safety and it leaves us feeling shut off from ourselves and the people around us.

With this new understanding of numbing from a nervous system perspective, we can return to the question: Where is the line between self-soothing and numbing? Or put another way: How do we know if the activity we are engaging in is a helpful, regulating glimmer or a destructive, dysregulating numbing device? The truth is, it's a fine line, and it can look different depending on the day and on the person. I believe we can find our line by being mindful of two things when we engage in potentially numbing behaviours: our intentions and how we feel in our body.

WHEN WE ARE NUMBING, WE ARE SENDING A MESSAGE THAT THERE IS SOMETHING DANGEROUS WE NEED TO HIDE FROM.

Identify your intention

We need to be aware of what our goal is when we reach for something 'soothing', because the line between a glimmer and numbing device isn't to do with 'what' we are doing, it has to do with 'why' we are doing it. A piece of chocolate cake in front of the TV might be a true glimmer and help your nervous system settle into regulation, but if you are eating chocolate cake in front of the TV because you are detaching from your feelings of sadness, you will likely wind up feeling numb and dysregulated. Ask yourself, *'Am I doing this to avoid feeling something else, or is this what I want to be doing right now for pure enjoyment?'*

Admittedly, identifying our intentions is easier said than done. There are times when our intentions are so unconscious and completely out of our awareness, that it can be difficult to recognise them. We might have no idea why we are pouring ourselves another glass of wine, or why we want to keep scrolling on TikTok. This is why staying aware of how we feel in our body is an invaluable tool.

Find your feeling

When you are drinking, scrolling, eating or engaging in any other potentially numbing activity, try to stay mindful of the feelings and sensations in your body and see if you can track which state your nervous system is in. Notice if you are feeling calm, present and clear-headed (regulated) or if you are sinking into feeling emotionally dull, disconnected, or on edge (dysregulated). This will give you vital clues about whether the activity you are doing is supporting you in feeling safe and regulated, or whether it's pushing your system into survival mode. If you find it hard to notice how you're feeling, taking a breath to pause and trying to put it into words – either on a piece of paper or in a note on your phone – can help you practise identifying your feeling in the moment.

It's easy to get sucked into numbing, especially when we justify our behaviour by saying things like, '*I deserve a treat*' or '*I just want to switch off*'. But when we turn to numbing devices to escape pain, the escape itself perpetuates the pain and we enter a dangerous spiral. When we reconnect with our intentions, our bodily sensations and our emotions, we can begin to tell ourselves the truth about what is soothing, and what is dysregulating. And let me tell you, the more times you choose to self-regulate with a glimmer – instead of abandoning yourself through numbing – the more habitual this act of self-care will become. In time, you may notice that instead of sinking into the sofa with a glass of wine and the remote after a tough day, you are choosing to roll out your yoga mat, run a bath or text a friend. The more we start to notice that these small acts of self-care create ease and joy in our lives, the more second nature they will become. Repetition grows into automation.

Spirituality

Another important type of numbing is the idea of spiritual bypassing. This is the use of spiritual beliefs to avoid dealing with emotional discomfort. The concept was outlined in 2002 by Buddhist teacher and psychologist John Welwood, in his book *Toward a Psychology of Awakening*. He defined spiritual bypassing as the use of spiritual practices as a way of *side-stepping* personal and emotional issues, or to belittle basic needs, and avoid 'developmental tasks' and feelings, under the guise of spiritual enlightenment.

When people fail to be honest with themselves about their feelings, their spiritual practices – like meditation, for example – can easily become vehicles of avoidance. They might try to 'rise above' difficult emotions, or 'transcend' the uncomfortable real-ities of being human before they have fully processed or made peace with them. And, in their efforts to sidestep their human-ness, they become disconnected from their true selves. Many so-called spiritual slogans simply tell us to 'eliminate negativity' or 'only focus on the positive' but this can keep people trapped in a realm of illusion and self-deception, which is ultimately a very lonely place. True spirituality isn't about escaping inner and outer truths, or severing integral parts of us. In order to become whole, we must try to embrace both the light and the dark side of what it means to be human. If you recognise you have a tendency towards spiritual bypassing, ground yourself in the knowledge that being human comes with its challenges and that you don't need to rise above difficulties or avoid pain. We can and should feel these emotions, too.

Numbing Anger

Anger is one of the most frequently numbed emotions, so it's valuable to consider it when discussing numbing. Anger often gets labelled as a 'negative' emotion. But anger in itself is not negative or unhealthy. In fact, the more we keep our anger bottled inside, the more toxic and unhealthy it becomes.

Anger gets a bad rap for a few reasons. Firstly, it's regularly associated with aggression, and sometimes the terms 'anger' and 'aggression' are used interchangeably, despite their very different meanings. The simplest differentiation between aggression and anger is that anger is a natural human emotion that doesn't necessarily have any specific action attached to it, whereas aggression relates to behaviour. Many people numb from their anger because they conflate it with aggression, and believe that it is a destructive force that needs to be controlled. But anger shouldn't be denied or minimised.

LIKE ALL EMOTIONS, ANGER PROVIDES US WITH VALUABLE INFORMATION ABOUT OUR INNER LIVES.

Our anger might be signalling that we feel violated, betrayed, unseen or unsupported. Or perhaps we feel rageful because our values are being challenged or something we care about is being threatened.

Another reason we might banish anger is because in childhood we received the message that our anger was unacceptable. Perhaps we were told – directly or indirectly – that 'good children don't shout', or that 'it's important to be agreeable'. Early lessons like these can become embedded in the mind and nervous system, and can play havoc with our ability to feel and express our anger. Sadly, children who disown their healthy anger may struggle to develop a sense of assertiveness around their own wants and needs, which can set them up for a lifetime of having their boundaries violated.

There is also a substantial amount of research indicating that supressed, numbed and ignored anger is a factor in many illnesses, including various forms of autoimmune diseases, chronic fatigue and diabetes. This is because the repression of anger is thought to lead to the chronic secretion of stress hormones, such as cortisol, that suppress the immune system. All emotions cause a specific, appropriate physical, hormonal response in our bodies. Remember, our bodies are incredibly intelligent and are always trying to keep us safe. When you experience anger, your blood pressure rises, your heart rate speeds, adrenaline increases in the body in preparation for our angry 'outburst'. The trouble is that, if this anger isn't released but merely squashed and held within – there's no bodily completion of this *natural* anger response. Therefore an imbalance may begin to build up, with these hormones released to protect us now loose in our system in the wrong balance, and they begin to deplete us.

Instead of numbing our anger, we need to understand it and embrace its power, and recognise that it can be constructive when it motivates us to speak up or make a change. The more we keep our anger bottled inside, the more likely it is that we will manage it poorly – perhaps with impulsive aggressive or passive-aggressive behaviour.

Women and Anger

Girls and women are often encouraged, sometimes in very subtle ways, to detach from their anger because it is 'unfeminine' or 'undesirable'. Women who stand up for themselves or set boundaries can be seen as rude or confrontational, when the same behaviours seen in men are seen as signs of power or confidence. Sadly, this is particularly true for Black women. The 'angry Black

8 Common Passive-Aggressive Ways of Expressing Anger

Being passive aggressive isn't about being malicious; it's often a strategy people use when they think they don't deserve to speak their minds or they are afraid to express their anger.

Hurtful teasing disguised as joking

Withholding positive feedback

Poor listening

Not returning calls, texts or emails

Chronic lateness

Poor follow-through on commitments

Inconsistent silent treatment

Backhanded compliments

woman' stereotype has undermined Black women's anger by deeming it as irrational and explosive, which has led many Black women to stifle, numb and suppress their healthy anger.

There is a common cultural narrative that women are more able to access their emotions than men; however, women are often limited to 'socially acceptable' emotional expressions such as concern, sadness or worry. There has been some cultural conditioning, which 'allows' women to be emotional as long as it's the *right kind* of emotion. We typically see crying as 'acceptable' but rage as not (with the permissible exception, of course, of the maternal angry 'mama bear' who protects her offspring).

All of us should have a licence to feel our anger. When anger is numbed or not attended to, it doesn't go away. It will usually only get stronger and will inevitably end up being expressed in unhealthy, potentially harmful ways. Bottled-up anger can be expressed outwardly in the form of aggressive behaviour but it can also be expressed inwardly and directed towards the self. That is, if someone dares not express their anger towards other people, they might redirect their anger and resentment for others towards themselves. Anger turned against the self can manifest as harsh self-criticism or self-harm, and often results in mental health challenges such as anxiety, depression or chronic shame. In her book, *Rage Becomes Her: The Power of Women's Anger*, Soraya Chemaly points out that, 'Anger is like water. No matter how hard a person tries to dam, divert, or deny it, it will find a way, usually along the path of least resistance.'

Reclaiming our anger begins with recognising that anger is like a warning light on our emotional dashboard, alerting us to a problem. Just like sadness or fear, anger is a valid emotion that communicates important information, and it is our job to feel it and decipher its message, rather than numb or deny it.

WHEN ANGER IS NUMBED, IT WILL INEVITABLY END UP BEING EXPRESSED IN UNHEALTHY, POTENTIALLY HARMFUL WAYS.

EXERCISE: WHERE OUR NUMBING COMES FROM

In order to heal from numbing, it is important to become curious about the origins of this coping strategy and to become aware of our beliefs about certain emotions. Being curious helps us develop compassion and acceptance, which are the foundations for change. Ask yourself:

- *When I was young, how did the adults in my life manage their difficult emotions like anger or sadness?*

- *When I was young, which emotions did I not see being expressed?*

- *When might I have learned to bury my vulnerable feelings?*

- *When did I learn to dampen my painful feelings and turn towards numbing substances or behaviours?*

- *What are the feelings I numb the most, and why might that be? (E.g. I don't like feeling anger because I find anger frightening, or because I have internalised the idea that it is unfeminine)*

THE HAPPINESS TRAP

The good news when it comes to numbing is that nobody is born with a trait of squashing down or hiding their emotions. As a baby, you didn't think twice before crying out for food or comfort. You had no qualms about expressing your big feelings, nor did you worry that you were inconveniencing someone else with your needs. But as you grew up, you might have received the message from the people in your life, or from society, that strong or 'negative' emotions were undesirable, and as a result, you may have started to numb or hide from certain feelings so as not to disappoint the people around you and to fit into society's expectations of you. There is an unfortunate by-product of believing that strong or painful emotions are unacceptable: you internalise the false belief that you are supposed to be happy all of the time.

It's a common myth that happiness is a natural state for human beings. Not only is this unrealistic, but it's also very dangerous. When we try to be in a sustained state of happiness, we cut ourselves off from our entire scope of emotions, and we fuel our compulsion to escape difficult feelings through numbing – because when a difficult emotion pops up, we think we're supposed to Whac-A-Mole it back down again and go back to feeling happy. The truth is, real happiness is not about feeling 'good' all the time; it's about having the freedom to experience all of our emotions, as and when they arise. The realisation that we *should* feel the whole kaleidoscope of our feelings is often a revelation for people in therapy, as described by Glennon Doyle: 'I did not know I was supposed to feel everything. I thought I was supposed to feel happy.' It is part of the full experience of life that we feel not only happiness, love and joy, but also jealousy, rage, shame, sadness, guilt, grief, despair, greed, and remorse. Our emotions make life meaningful and exciting; they help us connect with other people and they guide us towards what we really want and need.

How to feel your feelings

Hopefully by now you are starting to understand that reclaiming your whole self means reclaiming the emotions you disowned. Being free to feel spontaneous emotions without supressing them is a sign of emotional health, but it isn't always easy to turn towards our pain if we have a history of habitually numbing or avoiding our feelings.

It might sound odd, but the first step in learning to feel our feelings is to trust that we can *cope* with our feelings. Many people resist leaning in to their painful emotions because they fear that their emotions will destroy them in some way. They might worry that if they let themselves fully feel their sadness, shame, grief, or anger that they won't be able to manage – perhaps that they will never stop crying, lose control or 'open a can of worms'. When we indulge the notion that we can't tolerate our pain, we are actually siding with our inner critic. And this sneaky negative internal voice can fuel our desire to numb our emotions. First, it says, '*Don't get upset, that's a bad idea, just have some chocolate and you'll feel better*' or '*Don't bother getting angry. What's the point? You've had a tough day, you deserve to switch off and have a beer*', but then after we have indulged, it punishes us with harsh criticisms, '*You're so greedy and lazy*' or '*You drank too much again*'. Part of overcoming a habit of numbing involves trusting that we have the inner resources to cope with our difficult feelings.

I can assure you that your painful emotions won't kill you and they won't last forever, despite what your catastrophic thoughts might tell you. If we want to turn away from numbing and embrace our wholeness, we must face all of our feelings – the only way out is through. However, it should also be said that if you have spent your whole life pushing your feelings away, you might need to gradually build up your tolerance for feeling the hard stuff. Suddenly fully experiencing your grief, shame or anger can be overwhelming to your nervous system, especially if you have a history of avoiding your feelings or you have an oversensitive nervous system due to chronic stress or trauma. Many of us need to gently grow our capacity to internally feel safe when we access our pain in a process American therapist Peter Levine called 'titration'.

Titration is a term used in chemistry that refers to the mixing of chemicals in a slow, gradual manner. For example, if you combine large amounts of vinegar and baking soda together, you will get an explosion. However, if you add the vinegar to a small amount of baking soda, one drop at a time, you will find that nothing gets out of control – there is only a small sizzle and then it settles down. We need this concept if we often find ourselves swept away in emotional currents. Gently welcoming the emotions that we previously forced underground is how we can feel what needs to be felt, and reclaim our wholeness, without becoming overly stressed and dysregulated.

One way to gently welcome back and reconnect with the feelings we have suppressed is with a simple, research-backed technique called 'Name it to tame it'. The practice was first identified by psychiatrist and professor, Dr Daniel Siegel, who recognised that labelling our emotions can help them to pass. Identifying a strong emotion ('naming') has the effect of reducing the stress ('taming') in both the brain and the body.

Siegel argues that if we want to increase our tolerance for feeling our feelings, there is a specific way we can label our emotions. Sometimes we are afraid to label an emotion because we think naming it gives it power but, in fact, naming an emotion dispels the power it has over you. Siegel suggests that when naming an emotion, we should say 'I feel' versus 'I am'. To say 'I feel angry' has a very different impact than the words 'I am angry'. The latter tends to define us as an angry person, whereas the former helps us to recognise that feelings are fleeting. It may sound nit-picky, but when you say 'I am angry' you conflate your whole self with the emotion, which can make the emotion feel permanent and overwhelming. Saying 'I feel angry' reminds you that anger is not *who* you are; it's how you feel. Siegel suggests that the 'Name it to tame it' technique is also effective because it brings our prefrontal cortex back online – the part of our brain responsible for complex tasks, problem-solving and impulse control.

Another way to become attuned to our feelings, and gently welcome them into our awareness, is to notice the sensations in our body. Many emotional experiences start in the body before moving into our emotional awareness. Shame might be experienced as a pit in your stomach, sadness might be experienced as heaviness in your chest, or anger might be experienced as a tightness in the jaw. The ability to pay attention to the sensations in our body is called 'interoception' and it's an important part of reconnecting with ourselves.

EXERCISE: NAME IT AND FEEL IT

When I first started training as an integrative therapist, I struggled to name the sensations I was feeling.

Something that was transformative for me in learning how to identify my feelings was thinking about it in terms of weather: what is the weather like in your body? Can you check in and identify a sense of what type of weather conditions you may have inside? For example, I might feel there are 'storm clouds' in my mind, or a 'sunny brightness' in my heart. If you're struggling to put words to your feelings, try giving this approach a go.

Next time you're experiencing a negative emotion, have a go at naming that feeling.

Write it down simply: I feel _____

Then, make a note underneath of body sensations you notice. By building a record of your feelings and how these emotions are displayed in our bodies, we are strengthening our interoception skills and, in turn, becoming more closely connected with ourselves.

When we reclaim our emotions at a safe pace, we strengthen our capacity to work through our feelings without getting swept up in them and, as a result, we reduce our desire to numb-out. The beauty of being able to work through our emotions – instead of numbing them – is that it allows us to clearly see our *resilience*. There is often a common misconception that resilience is about never experiencing emotional pain, or that it is about 'powering through hardship', but this is how many of us wind up living in survival mode; feeling anxious or depressed. Resilience is about being able to *recover* from difficulties, not endure them.

Resilient people let themselves have a bad day, feel their uncomfortable feelings, allow themselves time to recharge, then stand up and try again. Knowing that we have the strength and ability to bounce back after feeling bad is incredibly powerful and is often what stops people from numbing-out. When we recognise that difficult feelings will eventually pass, we stop being afraid of our intense emotional world and instead of hiding from parts of ourselves, we welcome them all, and become an authentic fully formed version of ourselves.

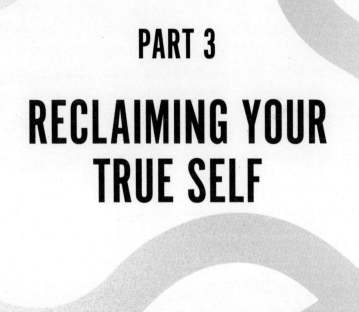

PART 3

RECLAIMING YOUR TRUE SELF

8.
SOFTENING THE INNER CRITIC

In Part 2, we looked at the things that get in the way of us being our true self: people-pleasing; perfectionism; chronic busyness; and numbing. These habits and patterns are unhealthy coping strategies. But they are learned behaviours and, therefore, they can be unlearned. Hopefully by this point, you have the tools you need to start to dismantle these destructive coping strategies and have more understanding of your habits and patterns, to make space to create a more fulfilling and authentic life. We can choose to make new choices that are more in alignment with our true selves and who we actually want to be.

This is where the tools we're going to cover in Part 3 comes in. Here we're going to learn healthier habits and strategies that will help you reclaim your true self, releasing you from the patterns that might have been keeping you stuck. We'll learn how to find your voice, set boundaries, reparent yourself, consistently practise self-care and understand how to better manage your feelings. But first, we're going to look at how to shrink your inner critic.

The inner critic is something we all have. In small doses, self-criticism can be useful; it tells us where we have gone wrong and what we need to do to make things right. But when this voice becomes meaner and more vocal, it chips away at our confidence, crushes our motivation and blights our self-worth.

The inner critic is that voice in our head judging us. It puts us down, compares us to others, attacks us with mean labels and induces fear and self-doubt. When we believe our internal bully, we can contort or hide ourselves in an attempt to feel safe and accepted, and make decisions that are out of alignment with our true self. I often find that when clients have lost their way in life it's because their inner critic has taken the reins. Ways this can show up in your life is feeling stuck in a job you hate, or not going for a promotion because your inner critic is telling you you're not good enough. Perhaps also you're refusing to be vulnerable in a relationship, or you don't go on that date because you don't feel like you're good enough. Remember, your inner critic doesn't allow you to see your strengths and positive traits – either telling you constantly that you're 'not enough' or conversely, squashing your vibrancy by telling you you're 'too much'.

There are many ways we can criticise ourselves. Here are four of the most common:

1. **I'm not … enough** (*I'm not successful/attractive/confident enough*)
2. **I'm too …** (*I'm too emotional/loud/selfish*)
3. **I should …** (*I should be happier/have moved on by now/not have done that embarrassing thing*). We can also criticise

our own thoughts and feelings and tell ourselves that we shouldn't feel anxious, jealous or angry, or that we should have 'moved on' by now. We might ruminate on embarrassing past events and find ourselves stuck in a whirlpool of shame and self-loathing.

4.   **I'm never …** (*I'm never going to find a partner/settle in at work*) And sometimes, for no reason at all, incredibly judgmental thoughts can pop into our head, telling us that we will never find a partner or achieve our dreams.

For those of us who regularly criticise ourselves, our self-critical thoughts have become our ingrained, habituated thinking for so long that they have become background noise; humming away without us even noticing. We might not even realise that we are constantly triggering the stress response and living in a state of chronic, low-level fear. An incessant inner critic can regularly push our nervous system into either an activated fight-or-flight mode, where we feel anxious or irritable, or a collapsed shutdown mode, where we feel unmotivated or ashamed.

In fight-or-flight mode, you might be flooded with anxiety-inducing thoughts and images: catastrophising and jumping to negative conclusions, feel like you're 'in trouble', or have to perform at 100 per cent. Or your self-criticism might be at the beginning of a self-shame spiral, which cascades into shutdown mode. In this case, one self-critical attack can bleed into another and push you further into a pit of despair, where you wind up feeling worthless and hopeless. You might make a small mistake like spilling your coffee, then criticise yourself by saying, *'I'm so clumsy'*, which might deteriorate into:

'I'm such an idiot'; *'I can't do anything'*; *'I'm bad at my job'*; *'I have no friends'*; *'I'm a complete loser'*; *'I'm worthless'*. It's remarkable how quickly we can plummet, leaving us unable to rationalise or see ourselves clearly.

The problem with having a harsh inner critic is that it triggers the body's threat defence system and pushes us into survival mode. Remember that in our calming, parasympathetic, safe-and-social system we feel calmer, and we're more likely to be able to feel confident and balanced in body and in mind. If we are pushed into our sympathetic nervous system too regularly, this contributes to our bodies being flooded with stress hormones such as adrenaline and cortisol, which can have a negative impact on all aspects of our physical and mental wellbeing. Understanding that even *a negative internal voice* can trigger this hormonal response is the first step to being able to proactively alter our internal behaviours for the better. As we have seen throughout this book, our nervous system's primary job is to keep us safe, and it jumps into action whenever it *perceives* some kind of threat. The stress response therefore might get triggered because you swerved to avoid a car accident, but equally it might also get triggered when you mentally attack yourself.

Because self-criticism can dysregulate our nervous system and gives us a felt-sense of danger, many of us employ our unhelpful coping strategies in a bid to feel safe. When our negative internal chatter pipes up we might try to feel better by launching into anxious productivity (busyness), or we might start imposing unrealistically high standards onto ourselves or others (perfectionism), or we might abandon our own needs and try to make everyone around us happy (people-pleasing), or we might try to mute our inner critic and dull our emotions with certain substances or behaviours (numbing). As we saw in Part 2, these coping strategies are all attempts to feel safe and regulated, but unfortunately, they tend to further dysregulate our nervous system and distance us from ourselves and the people around us.

ORIGINS OF A PARTICULARLY HARSH INNER CRITIC

We all have an inner critic, but its severity can vary from person to person. Self-talk tends to develop in childhood, based on how we were spoken to, as well as picking up on how our parents, teachers and family spoke to us, themselves and others. Our brains are like sponges and we often absorb the voices of the people in our lives into our internal monologue. These words may be positive, kind and supportive or negative, mean and unhelpful.

If your family were highly critical of you, your self-criticism might be particularly hostile or harsh. In these cases, the inner critic can be seen as the internalised voice of the parent, or in some cases, a sibling. Many of my clients use the same critical words and phrases as a parent or sibling would when they were young. It can be a lightbulb moment for people when I ask: *'Where have you heard this before?'*; *'Whose voice is this?'*

If you have a sibling, you may have also experienced cruel teasing and criticism from them, which was dismissed as sibling rivalry. But this dynamic can be the birthplace of a harsh inner critic and can have consequences well into adulthood. Squabbles, jealousy and competition are normal sibling behaviours, but when there is a repeated pattern where one sibling takes the role of the aggressor, it disrupts the one place a child is meant to feel safe – at home. And when the bullying is overlooked by parents, it can be experienced as abandonment and a lack of protection.

> DEVELOPING IN CHILDHOOD, SELF-TALK IS BASED ON HOW WE WERE SPOKEN TO, STEMMING FROM HOW OUR PARENTS, TEACHERS AND FAMILY SPOKE TO US, THEMSELVES AND OTHERS.

EXERCISE: WHERE DID MY INNER CRITIC COME FROM?

To try and better understand where your inner critic comes from, ask yourself:

- *How did my parents talk to me, and each other, when I was growing up?*

- *Did my parents judge other people?*

- *Were they critical and resentful?*

- *Were they kind and gentle to themselves and others?*

- *Were they understanding and supportive when I made a mistake?*

- *If relevant, what is my relationship with my sibling(s) like?*

Sometimes we can't quite pinpoint where our harsh or punitive inner critic has come from. Clients who were raised in unsafe, unpredictable or chaotic environments – for example, where parents are addicts or hoarders, but also parents who are highly reactive, emotionally explosive or unpredictable – often say things like this to me: *'My childhood wasn't perfect, but nobody ever explicitly called me a "f**king idiot" or a "lazy b**ch", which is what my inner critic says, so where is this coming from?'*

The reason why is because children in these environments will often turn against *themselves* to preserve their relationships with their parents. If a child grows up in a chaotic environment, with neglectful or abusive parents, they can blame themselves. Self-blame is a form of self-protection. Think about it this way: a child depends completely on their parents for survival, so if a child has grown up in an unsafe home, it can be too devastating for them to consciously acknowledge their parent's unfairness or cruelty. It can feel safer for the child to blame themselves and turn the criticism inwards. That is, the child imagines themselves to be the cause of their parent's rejection and this belief turns into self-talk that is particularly mean and cruel: *'I'm bad'*; *'I'm wrong'*; *'I'm unlovable'*; *'I'm worthless'*. These can then become core beliefs we hold about ourselves. What might have been an understandable survival mechanism in childhood can turn truly debilitating in adulthood. Further on in the chapter, we'll look at how to soften our inner critics as adults.

Self-criticism is not your friend

Harsh self-criticism keeps us disconnected from who we are at our core. The more we let our negative internal dialogue run the show, the more we lose sight of our positive traits and abilities. Softening the inner critic is one of the most import-ant steps on the path to reclaiming our wholeness, yet many people are reluctant to say goodbye to their negative internal monologue. Why would we want to hold onto something that is so destructive? Because sometimes we think we *need* our self-criticism in order to be successful. It's not uncommon for people to believe their negative self-talk is what keeps them tough, strong, motivated or ambitious. They fear that speaking to themselves in a kinder way will make them complacent. But the opposite is in fact true.

LETTING OUR NEGATIVE INTERNAL DIALOGUE RUN THE SHOW LEADS TO US LOSING SIGHT OF OUR POSITIVE TRAITS AND ABILITIES.

Here is a helpful analogy: If you were looking for a personal trainer to help you with a fitness goal, which of these trainers would you choose?

The first trainer shouts at you and calls you an idiot. They say, *'What are you doing? I can't believe you're doing a push-up like that – you look ridiculous! You're wasting your time even trying, you will never achieve your goal.'* Then they text you after the session to remind you of all the mistakes you made. The second trainer tells you that you're doing a great job and points out the areas where you can improve. They say, *'You're doing great – keep it up. That's your personal best! Next time remember to keep your legs straight'.* Then they text you after the session to tell you that you worked hard today and that you're doing a great job.

Which trainer do you think will help you achieve your fitness goals? It's the second one who will help you most. The

Here Are Some Hard Truths About Self-Criticism

Self-criticism doesn't motivate you to work harder, *it stops you from pursuing your bigger goals*

Self-criticism doesn't make you humble, *it damages your self-esteem*

Self-criticism doesn't drive you to succeed, *it puts you at higher risk of depression and anxiety*

Self-criticism doesn't support your growth and development, *it distances you from your authentic self* first trainer represents self-criticism, and this harsh approach will probably do two things: It will shame you and it will activate your nervous system's threat response. You might enter fight-or-flight mode, where you feel anxious or angry, or go into shutdown mode, where you feel hopeless and unmotivated. Either way, it's going to make you want to give up on your fitness goal and never see a personal trainer ever again!

By contrast, the second trainer will inspire confidence in you and motivate you to go back for another session. The second trainer is supportive, but they aren't just mindlessly complimenting you – there is encouragement *and* there is an understanding that skill development takes time. Not only is this more pleasant to be around – it's also a much more effective approach because it is *compassionate*. Compassion, as we are about to find out, is the antidote to the inner critic and it is an essential ingredient in reclaiming our true self.

WHAT IS SELF-COMPASSION?

Self-compassion might sound a bit touchy-feely and cheesy, but it's actually a very practical tool, which has a real impact on our nervous system. In short, self-compassion is the opposite of self-judgement, and it's central to silencing our inner critic. Self-compassion simply means giving yourself the same support, warmth and kindness you would offer a good friend.

There has been an explosion of research into self-compassion that demonstrates it's one of the most powerful practices that exists to change our physiology and benefit our mental and physical health. For example, recent studies indicate that self-compassion deactivates the nervous system's survival mode and activates the safe-and-social state. One study found that self-compassion reduces cortisol (the stress hormone that triggers fight-or-flight) and increases heart-rate variability, which is a measure of nervous system flexibility and resilience. It's therefore unsurprising that people who practise self-compassion have been found to show less depression, anxiety, rumination, as well as greater social connectedness and satisfaction with life. Developing greater self-compassion then is a vital tool for coping with and quietening our inner critic.

Dr Kristin Neff is a researcher and professor at the University of Texas. She runs the Self-Compassion Research Lab, where she studies how we develop and practise self-compassion. According to Neff, self-compassion has three elements: self-kindness; mindfulness; and common humanity. Let's look at each of these components in more detail and how you might be able to introduce them into your life.

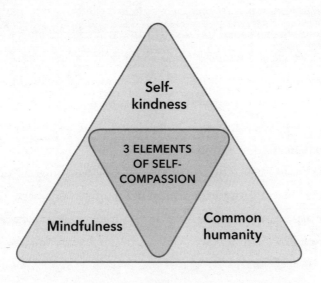

Self-kindness

This is being supportive and understanding towards yourself during times of difficulty, rather than being self-critical. Self-kindness sounds like: *'I tried my best even if it didn't work out the way I'd hoped'*.

Over-simplified and well-meaning advice about self-criticism is often to ignore your inner critic, but this is actually pretty unhelpful. What we need to do is turn *towards* the inner critic and try to understand its message. We need to show it, and ourselves, kindness.

If you were to ask your inner critic, *'How are you trying to help me?'*, you might find that, in its own weird way, it's trying to be a friend. It wants to keep you safe. For example, if we are tempted to bail on a social event because we don't feel attractive or confident enough, we can ask the inner critic how it's trying to help us. It might say: *'I'm trying to protect you from being hurt. If you don't go out, you can't be rejected. It's best you just stay at home where it's safe'*. Self-criticism can be sneaky like this because it can sound like a supportive arm around our shoulder and we can be tempted to go along with its bad ideas. If we were to indulge the inner critic in this example, we might avoid the social event, and, whilst staying at home might bring about some initial relief, it will ultimately lead to more anxiety, more avoidance and more self-criticism.

A compassionate and kinder voice before going out might sound like: *'I know you're feeling anxious about this event. You're not alone – plenty of people feel uncomfortable at social events. You always feel better once you get there; it's the anticipation that's the worst part. You can do hard things, even when you feel anxious.'*

There is a common misconception that being compassionate means letting ourselves off the hook, but the opposite is in fact true. When we show ourselves self-kindness, we make choices in our own best interests.

It's not always easy to find our self-compassionate voice, especially if our nervous system is dysregulated. If you draw a complete blank when you search for kind and supportive words, try getting out of your head, dropping into your body, and taking some steps to soothe your nervous system. Often, kind words will only start to come to us as we move towards a more regulated state. You might want to take a few deep breaths, have a bath or go for a walk – whatever you need to do to encourage an autonomic shift into a safe-and-social state. Once you feel more calm, try to imagine what you would say to a friend in a similar situation. Or bring to mind a person you know who is compassionate – a therapist, a grandparent or a best friend – and imagine what they might say to you.

Mindfulness

This is holding painful thoughts and feelings in balanced awareness rather than over-identifying with them. Mindfulness sounds like: *'I acknowledge that I feel sad but I know this feeling won't kill me'*.

Imagine you have arrived home after a social event and your inner critic has piped up. The first step towards being self-compassionate is to really notice how you are speaking to yourself. Your self-talk might be along the lines of: *'Everyone thinks I'm boring'/'Why am I so awkward?'/'People could see how anxious I was'/'No wonder I have no friends.'*

It might sound blindingly obvious to say, 'It's important to be aware of your thoughts', but many of us spend a huge amount of time barely conscious of how ceaselessly self-critical we are, and therefore completely unaware that we are causing our own dysregulation and suffering. This is especially true if your inner-critic is a continuation of what you heard growing up – many of us have completely normalised harsh criticism.

Dr Neff has one of the best explanations of mindfulness I have come across. She describes mindfulness as being aware of moment-to-moment experiences in a clear and balanced manner. She explains that mindfulness is the realisation of, '*Oh, I'm thinking this thought, I'm feeling this emotion, I'm experiencing this sensation*'. She defines mindfulness as 'a non-judgmental, receptive mind state in which one observes thoughts and feelings as they are, without trying to suppress or deny them ... At the same time, mindfulness requires that we not be "over-identified" with thoughts and feelings, so that we are caught up and swept away by negative reactivity'. What I love most about this definition of mindfulness is the reminder that mindfulness means not overidentifying with or exaggerating our thoughts and feelings. Yes, it is true that mindfulness means noticing, and not avoiding, our painful thoughts and feelings, but it also means not letting them run the show. For example, if after a social event your inner critic rears its ugly head, and you say to yourself, '*I was too awkward*', it can be easy to mindlessly slip into self-critical rumination and start spiralling and exaggerating our experience: '*Everyone thinks I'm weird*'; '*I'm completely hopeless*'; '*I'm never going out again.*' But when we mindfully observe our pain, we can acknowledge our suffering without exaggerating it: *'I'm feeling embarrassed and disappointed but it's not the end of the world. I know this feeling won't kill me and that it will eventually pass.'*

Common humanity

This is recognising that you are not alone in the mistakes that you make or the difficulties you might experience. Common humanity sounds like, *'Everyone makes mistakes'* or *'It's only natural that these things happen'*.

Dr Neff points out that a sense of interconnectedness is central to self-compassion. Recognising common humanity when you are being self-critical involves reminding yourself that all humans are flawed works-in-progress, that everyone fails, makes mistakes and experiences challenges in life. While this may seem obvious, it's very easy to forget that everyone suffers and fall into the trap where we believe things are 'supposed' to go well all of the time. The inner critic has a habit of telling us that we're the only person who feels the way we feel or worries about the things we worry about (trust me, you're not). Recognising common humanity might sound like, *'Everyone feels nervous from time to time. I'm not the only person who feels like this.'*

Self-compassion isn't softness

In my clinical practice, I find that people are often a little bit dubious about self-compassion at first. They are suspicious that self-compassion means letting themselves off the hook, making excuses, or that it will make them arrogant or unmotivated. But hopefully you are starting to see that self-compassion is actually the opposite of these things.

Just because you are being kind to yourself, it doesn't mean you are going to lie around all day watching TV and eating crisps. As Dr Neff points out, would a compassionate mother let her child eat ice cream for breakfast every day? No, of course not. Instead of allowing her child to be indulgent, she would acknowledge that ice cream is delicious and tempting, but then kindly encourage him to eat something more nutritious. Self-compassion inclines us towards long-term well-being, not short-term pleasure.

I used to be a smoker. I was actually a very heavy cigarette smoker for about 15 years and I tried to quit many times before I was successful. It took me a few failed attempts before I realised that my harsh inner critic was sabotaging my goal. When I felt a cigarette craving, my inner critic would convince me that I couldn't tolerate the discomfort: *'You can't cope with these cravings, they are unbearable; just have a cigarette and you'll feel better.'* When I listened to my inner critic and succumbed to the cravings, my critical voice would then scold and frighten me: *'What is wrong with you? Why do you have no self-discipline? You're never going to beat this, you're going to die of lung cancer and it will be your own fault.'* Just like the critical personal trainer we heard about earlier, my self-criticism only made things worse. It impaired my ability to self-regulate and made me crave the 'comfort' of cigarettes even more. One day, my therapist suggested I show myself more warmth and kindness. I was sceptical. Don't I need more willpower, more motivation, more 'tough talk'? It turns out I was wrong, and when I practised mindful self-compassion, I was able to quit for good. It worked for a few reasons. Firstly, after finishing my last ever cigarette I didn't deny my feelings. I acknowledged both the huge loss that giving up cigarettes was for me and the discomfort it caused – which validated and soothed my anxiety – but crucially, I didn't over-identify with my difficult thoughts and feelings to the point where I allowed them to let me off the hook (mindfulness). I also acknowledged that quitting smoking was one of the kindest things I could do for myself, that I deserved to be cared for and that it was short-term pain for long-term gain (self-kindness). And instead of throwing myself a pity-party every time I felt an uncomfortable craving, I recognised that quitting smoking was a challenge for everyone and that I wasn't alone (common humanity). I think the most powerful element of practising self-compassion while quitting was that speaking to myself with warmth helped my nervous system stay regulated, which was a gamechanger for tolerating the cravings and maintaining self-belief.

I truly believe that my final attempt to quit smoking was successful because of my self-kindness, not despite it, and it's been a powerful lesson that has stayed with me ever since. Mindful self-compassion is now something I practise whenever I face a challenge, big or small, and a strategy I invite my clients to try whenever they are suffering. It's incredible how much more we can achieve when we are being our own supportive best friend rather than our own worst enemy.

COPING WITH TRANSITIONS

On medieval maps, unknown and unexplored territories were sometimes marked 'Here Be Dragons' because it was believed that danger was lurking in these unchartered areas. Many of us experience a similar warning on our own internal maps when we encounter something new. Novelty can be frightening, and our threat response can get activated when we exit our comfort zone. Whether you are new to parenting, a job, a relationship, or a city, I want to emphasise that it is natural to feel some dysregulation in your body – the nervous system has a habit of confusing 'new' with 'unsafe'. During these times, it's important that we recognise our inner critic and grant ourselves some compassion, rather than judgement, about the discomfort we feel, otherwise we can easily fall prey to our inner critic's mean labels and anxious predictions: *'You're out of your depth; you shouldn't be doing this, you're going to mess this up.'*

OUR THREAT RESPONSE CAN GET ACTIVATED WHEN WE EXIT OUR COMFORT ZONE.

No matter how positive the change is, we are still disrupting our homeostasis when we do something new. Part of countering the inner critic and reclaiming our confidence involves understanding that it's normal to experience some discomfort when we are going through transitions. Growing pains are to be expected – they're not a sign that we aren't capable.

At the same time, we sometimes need to explore unchartered land at a gentle pace. In certain situations, it might be necessary to titrate (see page 164 for a reminder on this), or move incrementally, into what feels unfamiliar so that you don't overwhelm your system. For example, if online dating makes you anxious but you would like to meet someone new, try limiting yourself to looking at a dating app once a day, rather than endlessly swiping. Or if you would like to find a new job but the application process triggers feelings of fear and inadequacy, then start with applying for one job a week and build up from there. Part of growing and developing as a person requires tolerating some discomfort but if we do too much too soon then we will overload our nervous system, induce fear and end up in deep shame and failure.

We can also find ourselves in unexplored territory when we start to let go of destructive coping strategies and embrace healthier ways of doing things – particularly when we let go of the coping strategies explored in Part 2. Ironically, this can trigger the inner critic. For instance, if you choose to rest instead of frantically overwork, your inner critic might tell you that you are lazy. If you speak up about a preference instead of saying 'I don't mind', your inner critic might tell you that you are selfish. If you allow yourself to do something imperfectly, your inner critic might tell you that you are going to fail. And if you choose to feel a difficult emotion rather than suppress or numb it, your inner critic might tell you that you won't be able to cope.

Reclaiming our true selves involves accepting that we are bound to experience some discomfort when we open ourselves up to the unfamiliar, and resisting the urge to return to our old ways of doing things just because our inner threat detector is spooked. It usually takes a bit of time for our nervous system to adjust to the idea that it's safe to do things differently. A small amount of discomfort is a sign that we are growing, not failing. No matter what your inner critic says to you.

The Inner Critic Can Get Loud When We Let Go of Destructive Coping Strategies and Embrace Healthier Ways of Doing Things

When we choose stillness over busyness, *our inner critic might tell us that we are lazy.*

When we choose to put our own needs ahead of others, *our inner critic might tell us that we are selfish.*

When we choose to do something imperfectly instead of striving for flawlessness, *our inner critic might tell us that we are going to fail.*

When we choose to feel our emotions instead of suppressing them, *our inner critic might tell us that we can't cope.*

Instead of listening to your negative self-talk and returning to what feels familiar, practise some self-compassion and acceptance about where you are on your new path to reclaiming your confidence and authenticity. We often want instant confidence and comfort, but change doesn't happen overnight. It might sound obvious, but showing ourselves kindness gets even more important during challenging times. Self-criticism can spread quickly, but so can self-compassion. As Christopher K. Germer says, 'A moment of self-compassion can change your entire day. A string of such moments can change the course of your life.'

SELF-CRITICISM CAN SPREAD QUICKLY, BUT SO CAN SELF-COMPASSION.

EXERCISE: FIND YOUR COMPASSIONATE VOICE

Take a few moments to think about a behaviour that you would like to change. It might be that you want to drink less alcohol, be more assertive at work, or exercise more regularly. Then write down the compassionate words you need to hear in order to make that change. For example, 'You deserve to be healthy' or 'It's okay to ask for what you need'. This is about choosing kind and supportive words rather than self-critical 'tough talk'. If you're struggling to find kind words, try writing down what you would say to a friend who was struggling with the same issue.

Moving on to better things and a healthier way of living can also make us self-critical about our past. You might berate yourself for how you used to live: '*I'm ashamed of how I behaved*; *I should've known better*; *I have wasted so much of my life.*' Letting go of unhelpful coping strategies and spending more time in a regulated state can lift a veil, and we can begin to look back on our lives with fresh eyes. This can be an overwhelming experience, as we begin to judge and criticise ourselves. In this instance, quietening the inner critic involves forgiving ourselves for our mistakes and imperfections. Self-compassion isn't just about being kind to yourself in the present moment, it's also about being kind to versions of yourself that didn't know the things you know now. We are all imperfect human beings whose actions are the consequence of many causes and conditions. Most of the traits we dislike about ourselves are a combination of how we have learned to seek love and protect ourselves from pain. We need to cultivate compassion for every part of ourselves: the past; who we are now; and the authentic person we are becoming.

9.
SETTING BOUNDARIES

When people learn about boundaries in therapy it's often a surprising revelation. Many of us move through life feeling overwhelmed and resentful, completely unaware that we have the right to assert ourselves and communicate boundaries to others. Healthy boundary setting is something that few of us are actually taught, yet it's an essential life skill that can empower us to live our lives to the fullest.

In my experience, people tend to have boundary issues in two major areas of their life: work and personal relationships. At work they might take on additional tasks when their plate is already full, answer calls and emails out of hours, allow a chatty colleague to affect their productivity, let their holiday days go unused or do the work of two people. In their personal life, they might accept a friend's invite to go for drinks when they would rather stay home and rest, allow a family member to consistently give them unsolicited advice, let someone push them into sharing personal information they aren't comfortable disclosing, or allow a friend to vent at them when they don't have the emotional capacity to listen.

REMEMBER: WE HAVE THE RIGHT TO
ASSERT OURSELVES AND COMMUNICATE
BOUNDARIES TO OTHERS.

I deeply understand the struggle to set boundaries because it's something I used to have a lot of difficulty with. Before I learned to have healthy boundaries, my life was chaotic and exhausting. Being constantly in service to others meant that I was always overburdened and stretched too thin. I neglected my self-care, lost connection with myself, and carried around a lot of unspoken resentment. Even though I regularly felt mistreated or taken advantage of, I struggled to set limits with people because I worried that they would think I was uncaring, selfish or mean. It was scary to learn to set boundaries, but it changed my life in ways I could never have imagined.

BOUNDARIES HELPED ME RECLAIM MY
TIME, MY CONFIDENCE, AND ULTIMATELY,
THEY ALLOWED ME TO RECONSTRUCT MY
LIFE TO REFLECT MY TRUEST SELF.

Healthy boundaries have also allowed me to live more consistently in a regulated and calm state, and – much to my surprise – have deepened my relationships with others. I still don't always get it right when it comes to expressing my needs and my limits, and now and then I'll still struggle to set a boundary with someone, but boundaries, as we will find, are an ongoing practice.

Some Common Underlying Fears When Setting Boundaries

1. *If I speak up for myself, people will be angry at me*

2. *If I turn people down, they will think I'm selfish or uncaring*

3. *If I say no, people will think I can't cope*

4. *If I speak up about an issue I have, I will be rejected or abandoned*

5. *If I set a limit, I will sound petty or mean*

UNDERSTANDING BOUNDARIES

Boundaries are the limits and rules we set for ourselves within relationships. Boundaries establish, to both ourselves and to others, what we deem appropriate and acceptable and what we regard as 'OK' and 'not OK'. They allow us to separate ourselves from others and they help us communicate what we want, need or prefer. Healthy boundaries help us feel safe and secure within ourselves and our relationships (both romantic and platonic). We all need to set boundaries, but many of us have some underlying fears that feed our inability to set clear limits.

Some Common Underlying Fears When Setting Boundaries

- If I speak up for myself, people will be angry at me
- If I turn people down, they will think I'm selfish or uncaring
- If I say no, people will think I can't cope
- If I speak up about an issue I have, I will be rejected or abandoned
- If I set a limit, I will sound petty or mean

These fear-based thoughts are what drive us to be overly compliant and accommodating. Boundary issues can show up in different ways and in many different areas of our life, and they can sometimes have a different flavour depending on the state of our nervous system. For example, if you spend a lot of time in hyper-active fight-or-flight mode, you might say 'yes' to everything and everyone, and become anxious and burnt out.

Whereas, if you are more familiar with shutdown mode, you might feel small and invisible, and struggle to find your voice or self-advocate, which can lead to feelings of despair and hopelessness. It's hard to set boundaries when our nervous system is dysregulated. When we are in a state of balance, however, we are more able to access the confidence needed to speak up: it's easier to stand our ground, clearly communicate our limits, say 'no', and honour our needs. Boundaries can be quite chicken-or-egg: it's easier to set boundaries when our nervous system is regulated, and the healthier our boundaries are, the more regulated we will feel.

There's a common misconception that boundaries are about pushing people away, or about telling people what they can and can't do, but boundaries are actually a way to keep people in our life because they tell people what we will and won't accept. For example, rather than saying, *'You can't talk to me like that!'*, a healthy boundary is, *'When you raise your voice at me during a conversation, I don't feel respected or safe to express my opinion. If you raise your voice again, I will take a break from the conversation until we can speak more calmly.'*

WHAT ARE BOUNDARIES?

- Boundaries are a form of self-care

- Boundaries tell people what we will and won't accept

- Boundaries help us define and communicate our needs

- Boundaries are a way to create healthy relationships

- Boundaries help us feel safe

- Boundaries teach people how to treat us

- Boundaries are a way of expressing our limits

- Boundaries help regulate our nervous system

- Boundaries go hand-in-hand with a strong sense of self-worth

THREE TYPES OF BOUNDARIES

There are three types of boundaries: healthy; loose; and rigid. One way to begin to understand the three types of boundaries is with the garden fence analogy. Imagine you have a beautiful garden filled with different fruits and vegetables, surrounded by a fence with a gate. The fruits and vegetables represent your time, energy and resources. You tend to your garden daily and take care to feed, water and fertilize. The fence surrounding your garden offers some safety and security, keeping unwanted people out, but the gate allows you to let certain people come and go, and share your fruits and vegetables, whenever you please. This fence with a gate represents a healthy boundary: it's firm and clearly marks your land but there is some room for movement. People with healthy boundaries know what is their responsibility, and what is not, and they are comfortable saying no and asserting themselves in a clear and considerate way. Healthy boundaries are also flexible, and can be reassessed or changed given the individual person or situation.

3 Types of Boundaries

LOOSE	HEALTHY	RIGID
No fence	*A fence with a gate*	*A brick wall*
You have difficulty saying no	You are comfortable saying no	You have inflexible rules and restrictions
You believe it is your job to make everyone happy	You don't compromise on your values	You have difficulty being vulnerable or asking for help
You fear people will reject you if you don't comply with them	You are assertive in a balanced and considerate way	You avoid conflict under the guise that you are setting a boundary
You are susceptible to manipulation and accept mistreatment from others	You can be flexible without losing your sense of self	You keep others at a distance to avoid rejection
You overshare personal information	You share personal information in an appropriate way	You are fiercely private and protective of personal information
You are dependent on validation from others	You can be clear about how you want to be treated	You lack intimacy in your relationships and often feel isolated or disconnected
Example: *You say 'yes' to taking on an additional project at work even though you don't have the capacity, then you feel resentful*	**Example:** *You can say 'no' to an invitation, even when you know the other person will be disappointed, because you want to honour your need to rest*	**Example:** *You have a strict rule that you would never answer a work call after 5pm, no matter what the situation*

In contrast, having unhealthy loose boundaries is like having no fence around your garden at all. People just come in and steal your fruits and vegetables because there is confusion about where your land begins and ends. If we don't have clear boundaries, nobody knows where they stand, there are no guidelines or rules, and we are left feeling 'walked all over' and 'used' when people just take from us what they want. People with loose boundaries have difficulty standing up for themselves and tend to engage in people-pleasing behaviours because they define their worth based on the opinion of others, which regularly leaves them feeling mistreated and resentful.

At the other end of the spectrum, there are overly rigid boundaries. This is like having a tall brick wall all around your garden. Nobody can see over, there's no room for negotiation or flexibility, and the message is 'Nobody is welcome'. Rigid boundaries are equally as unhealthy as loose boundaries. People with rigid boundaries have strict rules and restrictions, with no flexibility, and are often fearful or controlling of others, typically because they have a history of having their boundaries violated.

Most people have a mix of different boundary types. For example, someone could have loose boundaries with their family, healthy boundaries in romantic relationships, and rigid boundaries with their friends. We can also oscillate between unhealthy boundaries that are too loose and too rigid. For example, you may have a pattern where you have loose boundaries and don't communicate your limits enough, then you feel overwhelmed and resentful, so you overcompensate with rigid boundaries for a while, and cut yourself off from people. Flip-flopping between having no boundaries – letting anyone in – to having rigid boundaries – letting nobody in – can wreak havoc with your sense of safety and connection. I agree with therapist and author Terry Real that 'If you're walled off, you're protected but not connected. If you're boundary-less, you're connected but not protected. Health is in the middle.'

WHERE DO BOUNDARY ISSUES COME FROM?

Nobody is born with boundary issues. The way we communicate and accept boundaries is largely formed in childhood and can be impacted by a few different factors.

Lack of boundaries as a child

Firstly, a lack of boundaries often develops if we didn't have a right to set boundaries when we were a child. Many people are surprised to learn that their issue with boundaries first developed because they had a parent who regularly ignored their limits. You might have had a mother who always barged into the bathroom without knocking, or who read your diary or text messages without permission. Or you might have been forced to hug family members out of 'politeness', even when you expressed your reluctance or discomfort in doing so. These boundary violations are dangerous lessons in consent because they teach a child to ignore their instinct to say 'no'. Parents who ignore their children's boundaries aren't doing so because they don't love their children; it's often a result of their own childhood experiences or emotional wounds, and this pattern can sadly get passed down through generations. Unfortunately, when parents disrespect their child's boundaries, they are sending the message to their child that their boundaries aren't important: that they don't have a right to their separateness or that they will be punished for having preferences. Early lessons like these become embedded in the mind and nervous system, and can play havoc with our ability to feel and express our limits. As an adult, we might find ourselves saying 'yes' when we would rather say 'no' because we don't feel empowered to set boundaries. Our focus, instead, becomes about pleasing the other person. We might engage in sex with a partner when we don't feel like having it, or let a colleague gossip about a co-worker, even though it makes us uncomfortable. Some people are so accustomed to having their boundaries violated that they don't even notice the discomfort that arises when someone oversteps their boundary, then later feel confused about why they feel angry or resentful. To reclaim our true self is to be honest with ourself about how it feels when our boundaries are crossed and to choose the radical act of speaking our truth about what we want and need.

Unable to express individuality as a child

We can also develop issues with boundaries if we weren't allowed to express our individuality or authenticity as children. In some families, there is unhealthy closeness in the parent-child relationship, with no emotional independence or separation between the parent and child. This is known as enmeshment. In healthy parent-child relationships, there is a balance between supportive connection and encouragement of the child's autonomy, but in enmeshed families there is no separation or space for difference. Parents in enmeshed families often use 'we' statements. For example, *'We like doing this'*, *'We don't believe in that'*, *'We are this kind of family'*. This confuses children into thinking that their emotions and opinions must mirror those of the parent and can lead a child to believe that autonomy and individuality are disloyal. Parents in enmeshed families are often easily hurt; they feel betrayed when their child doesn't want to spend time with them and often feel threatened or suspicious when someone outside of the family comes in and takes their child's time. In enmeshed systems, the parent may also blur the line between parenting and friendship and involve the child in adult issues or treat them as their 'best friend'.

It can be really tough to grow up in an enmeshed family. As an adult, you might not know what your needs and preferences are – let alone how to communicate them clearly – because you were never given the opportunity to discover your true self. People who grew up in enmeshed systems can easily slip into boundary-less and intertwined romantic relationships or friendships, where they ignore their own needs or assume that they need the same things as the other person. Rationally, they might know that expressing separate emotions, beliefs and opinions is important but their nervous system might feel otherwise. That's because merging with, and pleasing others, ensured emotional and physical safety in the past, and the thought of expressing individuality can feel threatening.

IN ENMESHED SYSTEMS, THE PARENT
MAY ALSO BLUR THE LINE BETWEEN
PARENTING AND FRIENDSHIP AND INVOLVE
THE CHILD IN ADULT ISSUES OR TREAT
THEM AS THEIR 'BEST FRIEND'.

Learned from our parents' boundaries

Another way we learn about boundaries is through observing our parents' (or caregivers') boundaries. If our parents didn't model healthy boundaries, they may have inadvertently taught us to ignore our limits. Children are like little sponges and they absorb everything that's going on. If your parents had loose boundaries, and you saw them habitually overextend themselves, neglect their health, or perpetually put other people's needs ahead of their own, you may have internalised the idea that it's normal to have no boundaries, or even that boundaries are selfish. Alternatively, you may have witnessed rigid boundaries from your parents. If your parents had few close relationships, enforced strict rules, or were quick to cut people out of their life if they didn't comply with them, you may have internalised the idea that you need to build wall-like boundaries in order to feel safe.

HOW TO SET BOUNDARIES

Setting boundaries doesn't have to be complex. I've broken it down into a simple, three-step process of define, communicate and maintain:

Step 1: Define

Many of us are so disconnected from ourselves that we struggle to even decide where to set our boundaries. So, the first step in using boundaries is to define them.

One way to become aware of our limits is to listen to our nervous system – our internal security system – and learn to feel a 'true yes' or a 'true no' in our body – A concept that I learned from Ellen Vora in her book *The Anatomy of Anxiety*. For example, when your friend asks you if she can borrow some money, how do you feel? Maybe you feel a *'no'* in your body. It might feel like some tightness in your chest, a contraction in your muscles or a knot in your stomach. It's as though your body is saying *'nope, this doesn't feel right'*. A *'yes'*, on the other hand, might be experienced as spaciousness and excitement in your body. Perhaps you feel expansion in your chest, ease in your muscles and warmth throughout your body. This might be your body's way of saying *'yes, I'm happy to do that.'* Listening for a true yes or a true no in your body might sound a bit woo-woo, especially if you have been disconnected from your bodily sensations, but it's surprisingly empowering to be able to take cues from our body. When we are in touch with our bodily intuition, we can check in whenever a situation arises, and listen to our deep wisdom rather than get swept up in anxious, fear-based thoughts.

Of course, sometimes we need to go along with things we don't want to do. We might agree to cover a colleague's work while they are on holiday because they did the same for us, even though it feels like a *'no'* in our body. Or we might say yes to dropping groceries off for our sick friend, rather than following our urge to stay at home. Listening to our bodily 'yes' and 'no' isn't about being selfish and only following pleasure and desire; it's about becoming aware of our choices, making conscious decisions and putting an end to the regular automatic yeses that lead so many of us to habitually deny our own needs.

Step 2: Communicate

The next step is to communicate the boundary. It can be helpful to use I statements like 'I will', 'I won't', 'I can't' or 'I need' when we set boundaries and it's very useful to stick to *facts*. For example, *'I'm afraid I have dinner plans so I won't be able to make it'* or *'I will no longer be the mediator in family disputes.'* Make it simple and to the point, with no over-explaining. Sometimes we nervously waffle on so much when we're setting boundaries, that people actually miss the boundary. More often than not, when people cross our boundaries it's because we haven't been clear enough.

Timing is also important when it comes to setting boundaries. *When* we communicate a boundary can be just as crucial as *how* we communicate a boundary. If possible, try to set a boundary when you are feeling as regulated and settled as possible. When we are triggered, we are likely to be reactive: we might angrily blurt out something that sounds controlling, reflexively say 'yes' to something out of guilt or fail to self-advocate because we feel invisible. When we are regulated, however, we can communicate our boundaries assertively and respectfully. Remember, healthy boundaries aren't about making a person behave in a certain way, they are about expressing your needs and limits in an authentic, considered and compassionate way, and the prerequisite is a felt sense of safety in our body.

Sometimes we are caught off guard with a request. If this happens then remember it's OK to pause, regulate your nervous system and consider what is best for you. This could take a couple of minutes, or you might need a couple of weeks. If someone says 'Can you come to my event next month?', it's perfectly OK to respond with, 'Let me think about that and get back to you'. One of the best phrases to have in your back pocket if you chronically and compulsively stifle your 'no' in order to maintain closeness with someone is 'Let me get back to you' because it gives you time to decide what's best for *you*.

Saying 'no' also doesn't have to damage relationships. In fact, saying yes begrudgingly is what damages our relationships because it makes us feel resentful. And let me tell you, other people can easily detect our resentment – it's pretty difficult to hide. I often ask people: 'Would you want someone to tell you "yes", and then resent you later?' The answer is always, 'no'. It might seem paradoxical, but expressing an authentic no is actually the best thing we can do in the interest of our relationships because being clear with people is how we build mutual trust and respect. The people I feel closest to in my life are the people who can communicate healthy boundaries, because I always know where I stand with them. I trust that they will be honest with me about their limits and their yeses hold more value because I know they really mean it.

Step 3: Maintain

The final – and sometimes most challenging – step in boundary setting involves maintaining, or upholding, the boundary. If you are new to setting boundaries, you may feel some stress and discomfort after communicating your needs, particularly if you sense someone is disappointed or inconvenienced by your boundary. It's important to remember that it's OK for your boundaries to disappoint other people – it doesn't mean you have done something 'wrong'. Feeling guilty doesn't mean you *are* guilty, and it isn't a reason to back down or retract your boundary.

IT'S ALSO NOT YOUR JOB TO MANAGE OR 'FIX' SOMEONE'S EMOTIONAL RESPONSE TO YOUR BOUNDARY.

If you say to your friend, '*I won't be able to come to your birthday dinner because I can't afford it, but I will join you for drinks afterwards*' you might get some resistance, especially if setting boundaries with your friend is new for them and for you. Your friend might express their sadness, confusion, disappointment, or even anger, but you are not obliged to soothe or fix their feelings. Of course, we want to set boundaries compassionately and it's OK to offer some reassurance if someone has an emotional response to our boundaries, but it's important to remember that we are not responsible for managing how people respond to our boundaries. We are only responsible for setting them.

It can be particularly challenging to stand our ground if someone is trying to intentionally guilt-trip us into changing our mind and doing what they want: '*But you're my best friend, you have to be at my birthday dinner*'; or '*I always spend money when it's your birthday*'. For many of us, this kind of pushback is really challenging – it brings up feelings of self-doubt, uncertainty and

Here are Some Helpful Mantras if You Struggle to Maintain Your Boundaries

I refuse to make my decisions from guilt

It's OK if my boundaries disappoint people

Boundaries are not a way to punish people

Feeling guilty doesn't mean I am guilty

My emotions and needs are important too

It's normal and healthy to have boundaries in all my relationships guilt, and can lead us to go back on our boundary. If that's you, remind yourself that setting boundaries involves tolerating short-term discomfort for long-term happiness and freedom. Listening to our feelings is very important, but when we are new to setting boundaries, our emotional reactions aren't always a particularly reliable compass. If you've spent your whole life denying your needs and letting other people set boundaries for you, it's understandable that some guilt will arise when you ask for what you need, and it will take a bit of time for your nervous system to adjust to the idea that it's safe to communicate the requirements you have for yourself. When guilt arises, practise some mindful self-compassion – feel the guilt, but don't overidentify and prolong it. Remember that feelings come and go, and they don't need to dictate our behaviour.

OUR EMOTIONAL REACTIONS AREN'T ALWAYS A PARTICULARLY RELIABLE COMPASS WHEN WE ARE NEW TO SETTING BOUNDARIES.

Finally, if someone's response to your boundary is a complaint, it's OK for you to gently end the conversation and agree to talk again when they are more emotionally settled. This can require some courage but it can protect us from retracting our boundary and complying with others out of guilt. When we retract a boundary because someone is disappointed, all we're doing is teaching people that we don't really mean what we say. And if we repeatedly do this, we effectively condition people into expecting us to always put their needs ahead of our own.

WHEN OUR BOUNDARIES AREN'T RESPECTED

Clients often say things like this to me: *'What if I set a boundary and they say no?'*; or *'There's no point setting a boundary with my mum; she'll just ignore it'*. Many of us have had the experience of finding the courage to set a boundary, only to have it trampled over, which can be frustrating and disappointing and deter us from setting boundaries again. But the reality is, we don't need anyone else's input in order to set or maintain a boundary. This is why boundaries are so empowering – they aren't about other people's actions; they are about *your* actions. For example, let's say your mother keeps turning up unannounced while you're working from home, and it's affecting your productivity. You might set a boundary with her that sounds something like, *'I love it when you come over, but it's not convenient for you to show up during the week while I'm working. Can we agree that you will come over at the weekend and that you'll check with me ahead of time?'* If your mother agrees, but then continues to show up unannounced while you are working, that doesn't mean you need to give up on your needs. It might just mean that you need to set a different boundary, which might sound something like, *'If you come round again unannounced while I'm working, I won't be able to answer the door.'* If this feels harsh, ask yourself what will preserve the relationship more: Letting your mother in but being angry and resentful while she is there, or making sure that the time you spend with her is quality time when you can be focused and regulated. As Nedra Glover Tawaab points out in *Set Boundaries, Find Peace*, 'For our relationships to improve, we assume that the *other* person has to change. We are unaware of the aspects that are within our control.'

BOUNDARIES AT WORK

As I mentioned at the beginning of this chapter, a lack of boundaries at work comes up a lot for many of us. It can cause us to work long hours, take on extra projects and prioritise problems that aren't ours to carry, all of which can lead to stress, burnout and long-lasting feelings of frustration and disappointment. Boundaries are essential if we want to break-free from constant work and exhaustion but many of us are afraid to set boundaries in the workplace because we worry that we will let people down, be judged, miss opportunities or be criticised. The truth is, you can have boundaries and still be a good employee. In fact, in my experience, it's the people who have healthy workplace boundaries that are the most successful.

People who set boundaries at work gain respect because they are showing respect for themselves. They also have better work-life balance, which improves their productivity, and they tend to live more fully in a regulated safe-and-social state, where they can effectively create, collaborate and communicate. Remember, when we are regulated, we are present, focused and patient, unlike when we are dysregulated, and we can be snappy, stressed or distant.

IT'S POSSIBLE TO HAVE BOUNDARIES AND STILL BE A GOOD EMPLOYEE.

Boundaries at Work Sound Like ...

'I check my emails between 9am and 6pm, I will respond to you then'

'I don't have the capacity to do everything today. Which task would you like me to prioritise?'

'I'm not comfortable discussing this at work'

'I don't check emails when I'm on holiday'

'Thanks for inviting me to lunch, but I need to run some errands on my break today'

'I can't help you tonight, I have plans with my family'

Four ways to set boundaries at work

Just like in any area of life, setting boundaries in the workplace can be tricky. But here's four steps you can take to start building healthier relationships with your co-workers:

1. Say 'yes' in the right way

There's a common misconception that setting boundaries is all about saying 'no', but this doesn't have to be the case. Boundaries are often about saying yes but with some honesty about what is realistic. For example, *'Yes, I can help you with the presentation but it will have to be on Wednesday because my plate is full today.'* Managing expectations and being open about our capacity is an essential skill in stress management and a powerful way to reclaim our time and our energy.

2. Protect your focus

If you find that you often get interrupted and distracted by chatty colleagues, you might want to set sound boundaries that protect your productivity. This might sound something like: *'Sorry, I'm swamped right now, but maybe we can catch up later?'.* If you are worried that you will come across as rude, ask yourself, would I find this rude if the roles were reversed?

3. Avoid over-explaining

People often over-explain or 'sugar-coat' their boundaries to avoid disappointing people but this tends to make boundaries unclear and it can leave people feeling confused. Try to make your boundaries clear and to the point, with no over-explaining. For example, *'I can't work past 6pm today'.* When a boundary is clear, we are less likely to be talked out of it.

4. Keep your time off sacred

If we want to have work-life balance and avoid burnout, it's important to have boundaries that protect our downtime. For example, *'I'm logging off for the weekend now so I will revisit this on Monday'*. These boundaries allow us to spend quality time with our friends and family and protect the time we need to rest and recharge. Boundaries that support work-life balance might involve taking all of your allocated holiday days, setting an out-of-office when you are taking a break or even limiting how much you talk about work when you are at home.

The five common boundary mistakes

There can be a lot of confusion about how to successfully set boundaries. This is understandable and if you realise you make any of these errors, be kind to yourself and remember you are practising and can try again next time. Here are five common misunderstandings and mistakes about boundaries, and what you can do instead.

1. Phrasing your boundary as a question

Sometimes we set a boundary and then when nothing changes immediately, we give up and assume we're wasting our time. One of the reasons people don't instantly respect our boundary is because we have communicated it as a question, when in fact, boundaries should be statements. Try to stick to the facts and use statements like *'I will'*, *'I'm not'*, *'I can't'* or *'I need'*. For example, *'I'm not comfortable with you making jokes about my appearance'*. If you ask a question, you're more likely to get into a debate.

2. Not setting a consequence

Often, when our boundary is crossed, we get angry but we don't know what to do or say beyond that, and the violation gets repeated. When setting boundaries, it can be helpful to explicitly state the action you will take if the boundary isn't respected. For example, *'If this happens again, I will walk away from the conversation'* or *'If you call me again when you are drunk I will end the call'*. Remember, boundaries are about communicating where your limits are, and what you will and won't accept. They are ultimately about *you*, not other people.

3. Forgetting that you can set boundaries with yourself

Some of the most important boundaries we will ever set are the ones we set with ourselves. Self-boundaries might be around the way we engage with work, our health, our self-talk, our money or our time. Setting a boundary with yourself might sound like: *'I will not look at my phone as soon as I wake up'*; *'I will not spend money impulsively as a way to make myself feel better'* or *'I will not use words like "ugly" to describe how I look'*. Honouring the boundaries we set for ourselves can be a radical way to reclaim our time, energy and self-esteem.

4. Only saying what is 'not OK'

Boundaries are about letting people know what we deem 'OK' and 'not OK', but we often forget to communicate the 'what is OK' part. For example, instead of only focusing on what is wrong, you could say: *'It's OK for us to discuss politics but it's not OK for you to shout at me when I have a different opinion'*. When we only focus on the negative, our boundaries can sometimes come across as rigid or controlling, which can make people defensive.

How This Might Play Out With Boundaries With Your Family

NOT A BOUNDARY	A HEALTHY BOUNDARY
The focus is on the other person's behaviour	*The focus is on the self*
'You always drag me into family arguments and it's driving me mad'	'I will no longer be the mediator in family arguments'
'Why do you always call me when I'm at work? It's so annoying'	'I can't talk right now. I will call you after work'
'I'm so sick of you treating me like a child'	'I appreciate your concern, but this is my decision'
'You and Dad argue too much – it needs to stop'	'I don't feel comfortable hearing about your marital problems – please find someone else to speak to'

5. Only focusing on other people's behaviour

People sometimes think they've set a boundary, but all they've actually done is call someone out on their behaviour. Since we can't control another person's actions, the focus of a boundary should be about *you* and *your* behaviour.

The most transformative, but also hardest, boundary to set for me has been protecting my self-care time. As a people pleaser, saying no to taking on too much has been so challenging, especially since I'm self-employed. I have to say no to certain projects and really honour my schedule by not taking on too many clients. Even on my maternity leave, I had to work hard to protect that time with my newborn.

As a therapist, too, boundaries are really important. They're a big part of the work I do – for example, I don't speak to clients outside of sessions, nor do I tell them about my personal life. I see them at the same time each week too, to maintain a routine and reinforce our professional boundaries. I also have a policy that I don't work evenings or weekends and I have a cap on the amount of clients I see per week. Defining and enforcing our boundaries is always going to be an ongoing challenge, both in our personal and professional lives, but it truly is a life-saving practice.

10.
REPARENTING

In an ideal world, our childhood home was a place where we received all of the physical and emotional nourishment we needed to develop into healthy, well-rounded people. However, many of us were raised in homes where our parents couldn't meet our needs, perhaps due to their own unresolved emotional wounds, financial stress, addiction, or mental illness. It's easy to get stuck feeling angry or sad about what was lacking in our childhood but, as adults, we have the wonderful opportunity to heal our wounds and reclaim our wholeness by giving ourselves the things we didn't receive when we were children.

It is true that our childhood is over and we can't go back and change it. We can, however, have corrective emotional experiences that allow us to heal our inner child and live more fully as an autonomous adult. Some people have corrective experiences in therapy, and, through a secure relationship with their therapist, experience some of what they may have missed in childhood. But we can also become a kind parent to ourselves and relearn to care, love and protect ourselves through small, daily practices. This is called reparenting. It simply means recognising the unmet needs of your childhood and giving those things to yourself now.

I must admit, when I first heard about the concept of 'reparenting' I was a little dismissive. My inner critic belittled the idea that I, a grown adult, had an 'inner child' existing inside of me that needed nurturing and protecting. I find this to be a common reaction to the idea of reparenting, particularly from people who were forced to grow up too quickly and become miniature adults at a young age. But reparenting is an incredibly powerful way to heal and grow, and reconnect with our authentic self. Reparenting looks different for everyone, but it generally involves noticing and honouring our needs, rather than habitually ignoring them. By reparenting ourselves, we learn how to make choices in our own best interest and reconstruct our lives to reflect our truest selves. Reparenting doesn't involve following any linear steps and it doesn't have to be complicated. In fact, the best way to reparent yourself is through small daily actions. These actions fall into three categories:

1. **Nurturing:** Taking care of your emotional and physical needs, and restoring your sense that you are lovable and deserving of care.

2. **Self-protection:** Standing up for yourself and setting boundaries, and restoring your sense that the world is a safe and protective place.

3. **Play:** Reclaiming your playfulness and spontaneity, and restoring your sense that it's OK to express your creativity and joy.

NURTURING

One way to reparent ourselves is through nurturing ourselves, which means taking care of our own emotional and physical needs. Many of us were taught as children to ignore our feelings and abandon our needs, and now, as adults, we struggle to identify and understand how we feel and what we need. We might get so caught up in busyness and hyper-activity that we ignore our hunger, tiredness or thirst. For example, maybe you don't use the toilet for hours because you're tied to your desk, or you finish some chores only to realise you're incredibly thirsty. Or we might be so focused on supporting other people that we fail to recognise when we need someone to listen to us, or when we need some time alone. Self-nurturing means identifying our feelings and needs, and then honouring those things through self-regulation and self-care.

> THROUGH REPARENTING, WE MAKE
> CHOICES IN OUR OWN BEST INTEREST
> AND RECONSTRUCT OUR LIVES TO
> REFLECT OUR TRUEST SELVES.

Self-regulation

Self-regulation is the ability to monitor and manage our nervous system states, emotions and thoughts. We've been working on this throughout the book. In Part 1 we explored how to regulate our autonomic states through the use of 'glimmers', which are the experiences, interactions and resources that help calm the nervous system and move us into a regulated safe-and-social state: breathing exercises; a walk on the beach; a favourite TV show; a massage; a cuddle with a pet. Hopefully by now you have started to identify some of your own glimmers and perhaps even begun making use of them when you feel out of balance. In other chapters, we have looked at how to monitor and manage our emotions and thoughts. We saw that by identifying and moving through our feelings, rather than running from them, we can soothe our pain and increase our resilience. And that through developing a mindful self-compassion practice we can soften our anxious and self-critical thoughts.

Another way we can self-regulate is by validating our feelings. When we self-validate, we reassure ourselves that our feelings matter and accept them without judgment: *'It's OK to feel angry'/'It's natural to feel anxious sometimes'/'I'm allowed to want time alone'/'It's understandable that I'm sad right now.'* Some people grew up with a parent who denied their feelings or who failed to acknowledge their feelings without judgement or expectation. Such a person often continues to deny their own reality, and has a hard time regulating their emotions because they have trouble accepting them in the first place. They tell themselves, 'I shouldn't feel like this,' or they dismiss their feelings as unimportant. Parents who deny their children's feelings often do so because they think it's the right thing to do – they don't want their child to be unhappy and they think the best policy for making their children feel better is to distract them from their unhappiness or to pretend not to notice when they are sad or angry. But this can make a child feel unseen, unheard or lonely. Reparenting ourselves through self-validation is how we can deepen our connection to ourselves and restore our sense that our feelings matter. When we acknowledge and accept the truth of our internal experience, and treat our painful emotions not as negatives, but as opportunities to learn about ourselves, we make space to think constructively about what to do with that feeling and, if necessary, take compassionate action to alleviate it.

Self-care

Self-care is doing things that take care of our well-being so that we can be fully present and engaged in our lives. Self-care isn't a justification for doing whatever feels pleasurable; it involves regularly checking in with ourselves and asking, *'How am I doing today?'/'What do I need today to take care of myself?'* Reparenting yourself with self-care might look like making yourself a nourishing meal, decluttering your space, making a dentist appointment, putting on sun cream, taking your vitamins, having an early night or wearing comfortable clothes. These may sound like small things but the more we take care of ourselves through these daily actions, the more we deconstruct any core beliefs that we are unlovable or unworthy of care.

Lots of us automatically insist that we have good self-care but there is always room for improvement, especially for those of us who are people-pleasers or live with a loud inner critic. When we reparent ourself through self-care, instead of asking, *'Have I been productive enough today?'*, we ask ourselves, *'Have I nourished myself enough today?'*. Instead of asking, *'Have I tended to everyone else's needs today?'*, we ask ourselves, *'Have I honoured my own needs today?'*.

In childhood, some of us didn't receive care from an unconditionally loving place, and affection from our parents was increased when we were 'good' and withheld when we were 'bad'. When we are loved for what we do, rather than for who we are, we internalise the message that we have to be 'good' in order to have our emotional or physical needs met. As adults, we might believe that we have to earn our self-care through working hard or doing things for others. If that sounds familiar, I want to emphasise that self-care is unconditional. You don't need to meet any sort of requirements in order to be deserving of it.

It might sound strange, but if you're struggling to get started with a self-care routine then try treating yourself like a toddler. Think about what a toddler needs to be healthy and happy: nutritious food; structure; enough rest; time outdoors; comforting words; physical affection; time to play. Adults need all of these things too. As you would with a child, incorporate these self-care practices into your life from a place of compassion, not punishment. Creating new healthy habits often requires self-discipline and accountability, but try to give yourself a bit of grace and remind yourself that loving kindness – not self-criticism – is the path to lasting change.

WE DON'T NEED TO MEET ANY SORT OF REQUIREMENTS IN ORDER TO BE DESERVING OF SELF-CARE; IT'S UNCONDITIONAL

Nurturing Self-Talk Sounds Like ...

I need ...

I would like ...

I give myself permission to ...

It is safe for me to ...

It's OK to ...

I'm allowed to ...

I deserve to ...

SELF-PROTECTION

Another way we can reparent ourselves is through protecting ourselves from harm. Some of us grew up in environments that were chaotic, abusive or dysfunctional and, as adults, we struggle to protect ourselves from people, situations and activities that are damaging to our well-being. We might find ourselves in a toxic relationships and struggle to stand-up for ourselves when we are being manipulated or controlled. We might drink too much alcohol, eat too much sugar or consume too much caffeine. Or we might allow ourselves to be repeatedly triggered by the news, or by certain people on social media. We are often completely unaware that we are frequently exposing ourselves to things that trigger stress responses in our bodies, let alone able to take the steps to protect ourselves from them. Reparenting through self-protection means tuning into our mind-body system and being honest about what serves us, then setting boundaries and saying no to things that are unhealthy. The more we act like a responsible parent to ourselves, the more we see ourselves as worthy of love and protection.

Here are some ways to reparent yourself through self-protection:

Curate your social media and unfollow people who repeatedly trigger your insecurities
If you are comparing your appearance, lifestyle or relationships to those perfect Instagram influencers, or there are certain brands that target your insecurities and make you overspend

or feel insecure, then it might be time to unfollow them. Remember: you are in control of your feed and you have the power to make conscious choices about who gets your attention.

Be mindful about what films, TV shows or podcasts you consume

Be honest with yourself about how your entertainment choices impact you and your nervous system. Do true crime podcasts before bed actually relax you, or do they put your nervous system on high alert? Do you genuinely enjoy reality TV shows or do they leave you feeling anxious or inadequate? There are no right or wrong answers here; it's about being true to yourself about what you actually find enjoyable, then making intentional choices about when and how to protect yourself from things that dysregulate you.

Limit your exposure to the news if it's making you feel overwhelmed

Staying informed is important, but being constantly inundated with images and stories about troubling events can shake our sense of safety. If watching the news is frequently making you feel anxious then find a couple of sources that you can rely on and set a time limit for how much you consume, and avoid looking at the news as soon as you wake up – we tend to feel more stressed in the morning due to a spike in the stress hormone cortisol within the first hour of waking. It can be tempting to check the headlines as soon as you wake, but it might be better for your anxiety levels to consume news once your cortisol levels have decreased.

Be assertive and stand up for yourself

Many of us are afraid that if we assert ourselves, we will offend or anger people, and be rejected or abandoned. But the alternative – letting people walk all over us – is a form of self-abandonment and can leave us vulnerable to harm. Protecting yourself in day-to-day life might look like expressing your preferences to an overbearing mother-in law, letting your partner know that their comment hurt you, or setting a boundary with a manipulative co-worker. Remember: you can be assertive without being rude or aggressive.

Say goodbye to unhealthy relationships

Spending time with people who are consistently critical, unsupportive, negative or judgemental can dysregulate our nervous system and contribute to anxiety, depression and low self-worth. Think about how you feel most often when interacting with the people in your life. Do you feel tense, anxious, deflated, withdrawn? Or do you feel safe, energised, free and secure? It can be painful to end relationships but sometimes it's the only way to reclaim your happiness and make space for relationships where you feel fully seen, heard, accepted, and able to express your authentic self.

Watch what you put in your body

Too much caffeine, alcohol, sugar or junk food can provoke a stress response in our bodies and send a message to our brain that something is off, as described in Dr Ellen Vora's groundbreaking book, *The Anatomy of Anxiety*. Protecting ourselves from sugar crashes, hangovers, inflammatory foods and caffeine jitters helps our nervous system stay balanced and restores our sense that our well-being is important and worth protecting.

EXAMPLES OF EFFECTIVE WAYS TO REPARENT OURSELVES BY SETTING IF/THEN BOUNDARIES:

- *'If I feel manipulated, then I will stand up for myself'*

- *'If I feel overwhelmed by the news, then I will take a break'*

- *'If I feel anxious, then I will limit my caffeine consumption'*

- *'If a brand on social media is repeatedly triggering me, then I will unfollow them'*

Play

We looked earlier at play, in Chapter 3. Play is a wonderful way to reparent yourself, by creating opportunities for your joy to be activated. Adult play is a purposeless activity that brings about joy and pleasure, and might involve dancing, painting, games, jigsaws, making music, pottery, rock climbing, or colouring. Play is an important part of well-being and can have a significant impact on the health of our nervous system, yet many of us avoid play because we tell ourselves that it is silly, unproductive or a waste of time. Some of this comes from societal pressure, and our culture's obsession with being productive, but for many of us, our reluctance to play stems from messages we received in childhood.

Our parents may have ignored some of our hobbies in favour of more academic pursuits, or we may have been told that we weren't 'naturally creative'. Or, if our parents never played with us, we may have internalised the idea that playfulness is childish, or that games are only about 'winning'. Alternatively, if we had parents who prioritised play and pleasure over their adult responsibilities, we may associate play with fear and recklessness.

Adult play is crucial to our well-being for a few reasons. We saw in Chapter 3 that play can help shift our nervous system into a more regulated state, and, over time, can even reshape our nervous system and strengthen our autonomic resilience. Play also helps us come into contact with elements of our authentic self that we may have suppressed over the years, and can be a healthy form of escapism if we need a break from our ruminating thoughts.

Reparenting through play might involve returning to known, feel-good childhood activities like building a Lego structure, watching a Disney movie under a cosy blanket, riding a bike, swimming and then eating a delicious snack, building a snowman or visiting an amusement park. Or, if your childhood had fewer of these experiences, reparenting through play might involve trying something you have always wanted to do: taking an art class; starting a scrapbook; learning to play an instrument; doing a creative writing course; or dressing up for Halloween.

It probably won't surprise you to know that people often feel self-conscious when they first start being more expressive, playful, creative, spontaneous or silly. What may be unexpected, however, is the potentially painful emotional impact of unleashing joy. If you find that you experience a profound sadness when you first start integrating play into your life, that may suggest that you need to grieve for what you didn't experience as a child. This is part of reparenting for many of us, and it's important to allow these feelings to surface without shame. You may also notice some anger coming up, which is a natural response to reflecting on the ways that your needs weren't met as a child. Try not to ignore or repress these emotions, and remind yourself that all emotions can illuminate a path towards healing and growth.

10 THINGS YOUR INNER CHILD MIGHT NEED TO HEAR:

Many of us have a younger part of ourselves that was never quite loved the way we needed as a child, and speaking to our 'inner child' can be a very powerful way to heal some of these childhood wounds. Repeat to yourself any of these mantras that resonate with you:

- *You are a good person*
- *You are allowed to express your joy and excitement*
- *From now on, I am going to keep you safe*
- *Being sensitive is a strength*
- *You don't need to be perfect to get my love*
- *I'm so glad you were born*
- *Your feelings matter to me*
- *I enjoy taking care of you*
- *You are not selfish for thinking about yourself*
- *You are so loveable*

Not many people have heard of reparenting, but it's becoming more and more popular. Some of us might feel guilt towards our parents at the idea of 'reparenting', feeling like it implies that our parents were 'bad', but the practice isn't about criticising the parenting you received. Instead, it's focused on *giving yourself what you need*. In most cases, our parents did the best they could with the tools they had, and so reparenting isn't about blame, but instead about growth.

11.
EMOTIONAL INTELLIGENCE

When people first come to see me for therapy, I always begin by asking them what they would like to get out of the process. They almost always say something about their emotions. Some clients think they are 'too sensitive' and would like to get better at managing their emotions. Others say they want to get rid of a particularly painful emotion. And some clients would like to improve their ability to feel or express their emotions. Whatever their goal is, the work we inevitably do together will involve some element of emotional intelligence development.

In its simplest terms, emotional intelligence is the ability to understand and manage your feelings, and to recognise the emotional experiences of those around you. Without emotional intelligence, we are often cut off from ourselves and others, so it's an essential skill to develop if we want to reclaim our wholeness and happiness, and live life from a more fully regulated place. In many ways, we've been working on building our emotional intelligence throughout the whole book, so this is the perfect chapter to end on and bring everything we've learned together.

6 Ways You Can Develop and Improve Your Emotional Intelligence

Embracing discomfort

Understanding the power of both/and

Staying clear of toxic positivity

Expressing vulnerability

Knowing your emotional triggers

Learning to listen

EMBRACING DISCOMFORT

One of the most powerful lessons people learn in therapy is that emotions are neither 'good' or 'bad'; they are merely sources of information, signalling something important we need to pay attention to. Contrary to popular belief, there is no such thing as a 'bad' emotion, there are only emotions that are more difficult to experience. When we judge an emotion like anger, sadness or jealousy as 'bad', then we are more likely to try and suppress it, which leads to more emotional suffering and disconnection from ourselves. As we saw in earlier chapters, running from or numbing our emotions doesn't make them disappear; it ultimately makes them more intense. It might feel good in the short-term to press mute on a painful feeling, but the relief is only ever temporary, and feelings will come back, over and over again, getting louder and louder, often in the form of physical symptoms, until we finally give them the attention they need.

> ALL EMOTIONS ARE VALID; SOME ARE
> EASIER TO EXPERIENCE, AND SOME
> MORE DIFFICULT.

The idea of welcoming all of our emotions may seem disconcerting at first. After all, many of us have been told to do the opposite. We're bombarded with the pressure to be happy, and have been taught that being strong means pushing 'negative' or 'bad' emotions away. But unfortunately, this is how many of us wind up living in survival mode, feeling anxious or depressed. To alleviate suffering we need to turn *toward* our

When You Say You Feel 'Upset' You Might Actually Mean You Feel ...

Angry

Sad

Let down

Humiliated

Disappointed

Shocked

Guilty

Lonely

Nervous

Fearful

Jealous

When You Say You Feel 'Fine' You Might Actually Mean You Feel ...

Happy

Optimistic

Content

Proud

Excited

Hopeful

Inspired

Confident

Thankful

Respected

Free

difficult emotions. In their book *Burnout*, sisters Emily and Amelia Nagoski write that many people experience emotional exhaustion and burnout because they avoid their feelings. They explain that emotions have a beginning, a middle and an end, and that we need to move through them to come out the other side, otherwise we will get stuck in a dysregulated state. They explain: 'Emotions are tunnels. You have to go all the way through the darkness to get to the light at the end.'

As you learn to face your feelings, you will discover that your emotional state is more complex than either 'fine' or 'upset'. Part of developing emotional intelligence involves increasing your emotional vocabulary and finding the right words for your feelings.

EXERCISE: FACE YOUR FEELINGS

Take a few minutes to think about how you're feeling and try to pinpoint words that more accurately describe the emotions you're experiencing (see pp. 236–237 to help you). Be as honest with yourself as you can but go gently – this sort of exercise is incredibly simple and effective, but also deeply revealing.

UNDERSTANDING THE POWER OF 'BOTH/AND'

If we want to successfully identify, understand and process what we are experiencing then we also need to be aware that we can feel more than one feeling at the same time. Many people live in a realm of black and white when it comes to emotions, believing they can either be 'happy' or 'sad', but emotionally intelligent people understand that it's OK to experience seemingly conflicting feelings at the same time. For example, when someone dies, you might feel both sad about the loss and thankful for the memories you shared. When you begin a new job, you might feel both excited for a fresh start and disappointed to have left your old colleagues. You might be angry at your ex but also miss them deeply. More than one thing can be true. Mixed feelings can be sometimes confusing, but the human experience is complex and we don't need to reduce our experience to just one feeling. When we limit ourselves to just one emotion, we deny important aspects of ourself, but when we allow space for mixed feelings to exist, we increase our self-awareness, improve the way we communicate our feelings to others, and reclaim our authenticity. Accepting that our emotional experience can be both/and – instead of either/or – also allows us to accept our emotions without judgement and let go of the pressure to 'fix' our feelings.

Both/and can also be a helpful concept to embrace when we are making decisions. A lot of us fall into the trap of black-and-white thinking when we need to make a choice, believing that decisions are either right or wrong. But this fails to take into account the complexity of real-life choices. Many people think that they need to feel 100 per cent happy with their decision to leave their job, move to a new city, or have a child before they take any action – they falsely believe that any doubt or sadness signals the 'wrong' choice. This often leads to anxiety and 'analysis paralysis', where they are so fearful of making

Examples of Both/And

'I am **BOTH** excited to be a parent, nervous that I won't be good enough'

'I am **BOTH** sad that the relationship is over, hopeful about my future'

'I am **BOTH** grateful for my job, sad about the sacrifices it demands'

'I am **BOTH** anxious about moving to a new city, curious about a new adventure' the wrong decision, that they let opportunities pass them by. Part of emotional intelligence is understanding that decision making can bring about seemingly conflicting feelings. Most decisions involve change, and all change comes with some grief, so it's natural for feelings of sadness to arise when we change or evolve. It doesn't mean you are making the wrong decision – it means you are human.

STAYING CLEAR OF TOXIC POSITIVITY

Toxic positivity is the belief that a person, despite their emotional pain or difficult situation, should only strive to have a positive outlook. It's putting a positive spin on all experiences, no matter how bad they are with phrases like, *'look on the bright side'* and *'good vibes only'*. Toxic positivity is damaging to ourselves and our relationships because it denies and minimises our (or others) genuine feelings. Toxic positivity can come from the external pressure to be happy all the time, but it can also come from a place of fear, or from a perceived lack of safety. The unconscious thinking is: *'I'll be safe and happy if I just stay positive'*. The problem with this approach is that when we refuse to acknowledge the negative, we are stifling our authenticity. And worse, we end up feeling a lot of shame and discouragement when we run into reality.

If you notice that your automatic response to challenges is to silence negativity and look straight for the silver lining, pause and ask yourself, *'Is this helping me?'/'Is the pressure I'm putting on myself to be positive all the time making me feel anxious and ashamed?'/'Am I silencing my emotions before I have processed them?'/ 'Is my obsession with feeling happy stopping me from showing up as I truly am?'*

Moving away from toxic positivity doesn't mean abandoning optimism; it means recognising the distinction between toxic positivity and realistic optimism. Toxic positivity forces us to suppress difficult emotions, whereas realistic optimism recognises that things in life can be hard, and that it's possible to work through them. Toxic positivity says, *'Don't dwell on the negative,'* but realistic optimism makes space for both reality and hope, and says, *'What are the issues and how can I move through them?'*

Expressing vulnerability

'Share your vulnerability' may sound cringey but trust me, vulnerability is essential if you want to deepen your relationship with yourself and the people you care about. At its most concrete, vulnerability involves sharing the true parts of ourselves that we fear may result in rejection or judgement. Vulnerability might be telling someone that you feel depressed. It might be telling someone that they have done something to upset you. Or it might be telling someone that you are attracted to them. Vulnerability involves putting ourselves 'out there' and it can be scary, uncomfortable or even risky, but it's a risk worth taking if we want to reclaim our happiness. Vulnerability is the path to authentic living, and absolutely necessary if we want to develop emotional intelligence and show up in the world as our truest self, yet many of us hide our vulnerability for the following reasons:

Toxic Positivity vs Realistic Optimism

TOXIC POSITIVITY

REALISTIC OPTIMISM

'Everything will be fine as long as I think positive' ➡ 'I'm going through something difficult right now, and it's taking its toll, but I know I will come out the other side of this'

'Failure is not an option' ➡ 'I will do my best but if things don't go perfectly, I will learn and grow'

'I don't dwell on the negative – it's positive vibes only' ➡ 'There will be some challenges ahead, but I trust that I have all the tools and resources I need to cope'

- *'If I tell people how I feel I will be burdening them with my problems'*
- *'If I show people my true self I will be shamed or rejected'*
- *'If I express my emotions I will met with anger'*
- *'If I'm vulnerable I will be viewed as weak'*

The avoidance of vulnerability doesn't just happen on its own. It's a learned behaviour that often comes as a reaction to having our feelings dismissed, ignored or ridiculed in the past. You may have had parents who told you to *'stop being so sensitive'* when you expressed your feelings, or you may have had someone tell you to *'just get over it'* when you opened up about an issue. These experiences can become embedded in our mind and our body, and we can start to feel anxious or unsafe at just the thought of telling someone how we feel. If this rings true for you, then you might need to express your vulnerability at a gentle pace so as to not overwhelm your system, but equally, don't allow the discomfort you feel keep you hidden inside your shell. Part of growing and developing as a person requires being open to the unfamiliar and tolerating small amounts of discomfort.

Vulnerability might be daunting but if we suppress or hide the true parts of ourselves, we can really struggle to have healthy, happy relationships. Invulnerability often makes us feel lonely, unknown and misunderstood. Because if we are always acting 'strong', we can inadvertently push people away – after all, it's difficult to relate to 'invincibility'. On the other hand, when we express our vulnerability, we are more likely to be perceived as authentic, honest and relatable. People appreciate vulnerability. When we're honest with others about our feelings, it conveys to them that we like and trust them and it gives them the opportunity to help and support us, which can add depth and meaning to our relationships. I've seen many people end relationships because the connection felt boring, stale or shallow, but often what was missing was vulnerability. Sometimes all it takes for a relationship to re-ignite or deepen is for one person to have the courage to share something that feels vulnerable.

> BEING OPEN TO THE UNFAMILIAR AND TOLERATING SMALL AMOUNTS OF DISCOMFORT IS NECESSARY, AND PART OF GROWING AND DEVELOPING AS A PERSON.

Admittedly, it's important to be vulnerable with the *right* people. Healthy vulnerability means opening up to people we trust, and recognising that it's OK to hide things from people with whom we don't feel safe. It's true that emotional intelligence involves expressing ourselves without inhibition, but it also involves being discerning about who we share our vulnerabilities with. Pouring our heart out to the wrong people is a sign of poor boundaries and can lead to more dysregulation, more emotional pain, and more disconnection.

KNOWING YOUR EMOTIONAL TRIGGERS

Being aware of your emotional triggers is essential to emotional intelligence. We saw in Chapter 2 that an emotional trigger is anything – including places, experiences or events – that sparks

The Truth About Expressing Vulnerability

COMMON REASONS PEOPLE AVOID EXPRESSING THEIR VULNERABILITY

THE TRUTH ABOUT VULNERABILITY

'If I tell people how I feel, I will be burdening them with my problems'

'Vulnerability deepens my relationships because it conveys that I like and trust the person I'm opening up to'

'If I show people my true self, I will be shamed or rejected'

'Hiding my vulnerability and always acting "strong" can push people away and leave me feeling lonely '

'If I express my emotions, I will be met with anger'

'People appreciate vulnerability, and, when I'm honest about my feelings, I get the connection and support that I need'

'If I'm vulnerable, I will be viewed as weak'

'When I express my vulnerability, I'm more likely to be perceived as authentic, honest and relatable' an intense emotional reaction, regardless of your current mood. It can feel like you're having a big emotional reaction that is disproportionate to what is actually going on. For example, maybe your colleague makes a comment that might not be a huge deal to someone else, but it totally destabilises you for the rest of the day. You might feel anxious, guilty, angry or sad but not really know why. As adults we typically become triggered by experiences that are reminiscent of old painful feelings. You might get triggered because you felt ignored, blamed, trapped, manipulated, judged, unheard, controlled, unsupported or helpless. It's like an old wound has been reopened and we are experiencing past pain in the present moment.

When we experience a trigger, our body kicks off a complex process of self-protection that readies us for fight, flight or shut-down. Our adrenaline spikes and stress hormones like cortisol run through our body and brain. When our stress hormones are released, we often lose touch with our healthy coping skills and succumb to reacting rather than responding, which is why it can be helpful to have some self-soothing strategies in your back pocket:

Here are 4 ways to self-regulate when you are triggered

1. **A deep sigh:** When you feel like your emotions are about to set off on a rollercoaster ride, take a few moments to slow down and do some deep sighs to calm your body. A deep sigh is your body-brain's natural way to release tension and reset your nervous system. When your exhale is even a few counts longer than your inhale, you release tension and prompt the body to 'switch off' survival mode (fight-or-flight or shutdown) and 'switch on' safe-and-social mode.

2. **Take a break:** It can be difficult to be objective when
    we are triggered, so remember that it's OK to step away
    for a moment to let yourself calm down. You can end
    a conversation, put down your phone or walk away
    from your computer. Taking a break can be immensely
    clarifying because it allows us to regulate, and it can
    prevent a counterproductive overreaction, such as
    shouting at someone or saying something hurtful that
    you later regret.

3. **Do some journaling:** When we are triggered, our
    thoughts can run riot in our head so it can be useful to
    give them a place to live. Journaling can help us release
    stuck emotions and make sense of our thoughts and
    feelings. Just write whatever comes to mind – there is
    no right or wrong way to journal and you don't need
    to follow any certain structure. Try to write without
    censoring yourself and remember that your journal is
    for your eyes only.

4. **Accept your feelings:** Be gentle with yourself and try to
    stay as non-judgemental as possible about your feelings.
    Often our triggers give us an opportunity to do some
    more grieving or to heal some things from the past
    that need to be dealt with. As the famous saying from
    American psychologist Carl Rogers goes: 'The curious
    paradox is that when I accept myself just as I am, then
    I can change'.

Learning to Listen

The final part of emotional intelligence involves being able to understand other people's emotional experiences, and this requires good listening skills. Genuine listening is a wonderful gift. It helps us connect, understand and empathise with other people, yet few of us know how to do it properly. Sometimes listening is hard because it can feel almost impossible to get out of our heads and stay focused on the other person. Or it can be tempting to offer advice – especially when someone we care about is struggling and we want to help them.

MOST OF THE TIME PEOPLE DON'T WANT TO BE TOLD WHAT TO DO OR HEAR YOUR OPINION; THEY JUST WANT TO FEEL TRULY SEEN, HEARD AND UNDERSTOOD.

There are two key elements to being a good listener: being fully present; and being agenda free.

Being fully present means putting your phone away and trying to fully focus on the other person. Pay attention to their body language and show that you are genuinely interested by asking open questions. It can be tempting to jump in and complete other people's sentences, but being a good listener means being patient and allowing people to find their own words and speak at their own pace. A good way to show someone that you have truly heard them is by mirroring them – which means repeating back their important thoughts and feelings using their own language.

The other element to being a good listener is being agenda free, which means putting aside your own wants, needs and opinions. When we have an agenda, we tend to be formulating our response rather than processing what the other person is saying, which can make people feel unheard and become defensive. Being a good listener isn't about knowing exactly how to reply: it's about knowing exactly what the other person is saying.

EXERCISE: **REFLECT BACK**

A skill that therapists learn is to occasionally summarise, or 'reflect back' what someone has said to show that they understand it. This is a technique that can be transformative in our everyday conversations and relationships. For example, you might say: *'Sounds like you're really frustrated'*; *'You felt misunderstood'*; or *'Sounds like you're saying you've tried everything you can'*. This helps the other person feel validated and understood, and it also allows you to check your understanding of what is being communicated and be corrected by the other person if needed.

Practice makes perfect when it comes to being a good listener, so try spending a day summarising or reflecting back the main points of a conversation or meeting. It might feel awkward at first, but it really shows people that you've been paying attention and helps them feel truly heard.

CONCLUSION:
THE JOURNEY HOME

We have arrived at the end of this book but your journey does not end here – it will continue beyond these pages. Reconnecting with your true self is an ongoing process, and your next step is to use the insights and tools in this book to support you on your path home to who you intrinsically are.

I hope this book has demonstrated to you that the way home is through harnessing the power of the mind *and* body. Remember: **your nervous system is on your side, and once you develop the ability to listen to its wisdom, you can allow it to guide you, keep you safe and steer you back on course whenever you lose your way.**

The more we listen to our internal truths, the safer we feel, and the less tightly we cling to our destructive coping strategies. When we drop our defences, we can begin to befriend the parts of us that we've been exhausting ourselves trying to run and hide from, and discover new, healthier ways to manage our distress. Letting go of people-pleasing, chronic busyness, numbing or perfectionism as attempts to feel safe and worthy, is how we reclaim who we are at our core and tell ourselves the truth about – and honour – what we need. It's a chicken-and-egg process: the more regulated we are, the easier it is to make choices that best serve us, and the more we make choices that best serve us, the more regulated we are.

EACH STEP BUILDS ON THE ONE
BEFORE IT UNTIL WE EVENTUALLY WAKE
UP ONE DAY AND REALISE THAT WE
HAVE RECONSTRUCTED A LIFE THAT
WE NO LONGER NEED TO REGULARLY
ESCAPE FROM.

Reclaiming our true selves isn't about being happy, calm and regulated all the time. It's about having the wisdom to understand that life can be turbulent at times but trusting that we have the tools to not only survive, but to bounce back better than ever. Our job is to listen. To remain mindful. To respond to our changing states with curiosity and compassion.

Like building a new muscle for weightlifting, growth doesn't happen in one big push, but in the small moments that build up in time. We reclaim ourselves when:

- We choose to say how we feel instead of saying 'I'm fine'
- We choose to let the sun shine on our face in the morning instead of our phone screen
- We choose to tell a friend that we don't have the emotional capacity to listen to them

- We choose to play, even when there are still items on our to-do list
- We choose to be alone with our own thoughts, instead of reaching for a distraction
- We choose to speak-up about a preference when we would normally say 'I don't mind'
- We choose to validate a painful feeling instead of numbing it with alcohol

You will inevitably experience some growing pains when you start to do things differently. A small amount of discomfort is a sign that you are growing stronger and more resilient, but remember that it's important to find the right degree of challenge for your mind-body system so as to not become overwhelmed. This requires self-compassion and patience, and it's essential if you want to make positive, lasting change. When you mindfully and gently peel back your layers of self-protection and reveal your authentic self, you will find that the world is a much more exciting and welcoming place to be.

REFERENCES AND FURTHER READING

Listed in order or appearance within the text

PART 1

1. Porges, S. (2011). *The Polyvagal Theory: Neurophysiological foundations of emotions, attachment, communication, and self-regulation.* W. W. Norton & Co.

2. Dana, D. and Porges, S. (2018). *The Polyvagal Theory in Therapy.* 1st ed. Norton Professional Books.

3. Levine, Peter A. (1997). *Waking the Tiger: Healing Trauma: The Innate Capacity to Transform Overwhelming Experiences.* North Atlantic Books.

4. Dana, D. (2021). *Anchored: How to Befriend Your Nervous System Using Polyvagal Theory.* Sounds True Inc.

5. Stellar, J.E., John-Henderson, N., Anderson, C.L., Gordon, A.M., McNeil, G.D., Keltner, D. 'Positive affect and markers of inflammation: discrete positive emotions predict lower levels of inflammatory cytokines'. *Emotion.* 2015 Apr, 15 (2):129-33.

6. Piff, P.K., Dietze, P., Feinberg, M., Stancato, D.M., & Keltner, D. (2015). 'Awe, the small self, and prosocial behavior', in *Journal of Personality and Social Psychology*, 108(6), 883–899.

7. Rudd M., Vohs K.D., Aaker J. 'Awe expands people's perception of time, alters decision making, and enhances well-being', in *Psychol Sci.* 2012 Oct 1;23(10):1130–6.

8. Shiota, M., Keltner, D. & Mossmann, A. (2007) 'The nature of awe: Elicitors, appraisals, and effects on self-concept', in *Cognition and Emotion*, 21:5, 944–963.

9. Ewert, Alan & Chang, Yun. (2018). 'Levels of Nature and Stress Response', in *Behavioral Sciences*. 8. 49. 10.3390/bs8050049.

10. Maas, J., Spreeuwenberg, P., van Winsum-Westra, M., Verheij, R. A., Vries, S., & Groenewegen, P. P. (2009). 'Is Green Space in the Living Environment Associated with People's Feelings of Social

Safety?' in *Environment and Planning A: Economy and Space*, 41(7), 1763–1777.

11. Van den Berg, M.M.H.E.; Maas, J.; Muller, R.; Braun, A.; Kaandorp, W.; Van Lien, R.; Van Poppel, M.N.M.; Van Mechelen, W.; Van den Berg, A.E. 'Autonomic Nervous System Responses to Viewing Green and Built Settings: Differentiating Between Sympathetic and Parasympathetic Activity', *int. J. Environ. Res. Public Health* 2015, *12*, 15860–15874.

12. Kahn, P. H., Jr., Severson, R. L., & Ruckert, J. H. (2009). 'The human relation with nature and technological nature', in *Current Directions in Psychological Science*, 18(1), 37–42.

13. Porges, S. (2015). 'Play as Neural Exercise: Insights from the Polygaval Theory', in D. Pearce-McCall (ed.), *The Power of Play for Mind Brain Health* (pp. 3-7).

PART 2

1. Walker, P. (2013). *Complex PTSD: From Surviving to Thriving: A Guide and Map for Recovering From Childhood Trauma*. Lafayette.

2. Brown, B. (2020). *The Gifts of Imperfection: Let Go of Who You Think You're Supposed to be and Embrace Who You Are*. Vermilion.

3. Aronson, E., Willerman, B., & Floyd, J. (1966). 'The effect of a pratfall on increasing interpersonal attractiveness', in *Psychonomic Science*, 4(6), 227–228.

4. Clance, P. and Imes, S. (1978). 'The imposter phenomenon in high achieving women: Dynamics and therapeutic intervention', in *Psychotherapy: Theory, Research & Practice*, 15(3), pp.241-247.

5. Hibberd, J. (2019). *The Imposter Cure: how to stop feeling like a fraud and escape the mind-trap of imposter syndrome*. Aster.

6. Winnicott, Donald W. (1956). 'Primary maternal preoccupation', in *Collected papers, through paediatrics to psychoanalysis* (pp. 300-305). London: Tavistock Publications, 1958.

7. Koretz, J. (2019). *What Happens When Your Career Becomes Your Whole Identity?* Harvard Business Review.

8. Dana, D. (2021). *Anchored: How to Befriend Your Nervous System Using Polyvagal Theory*. Sounds True Inc.

9. Tolle, E. (2016). *Stillness Speaks*. Yellow Kite.

10. Dalton-Smith, S. (2019). *Sacred Rest: Recover Your Life, Renew Your Energy, Restore Your Sanity*. Time Warner Trade Publishing.

11. Mate, D. G. (2018). *In the Realm of Hungry Ghosts*. Vermilion.
12. Brown, B. (2018). *Dare to Lead*. Vermilion.
13. Welwood, J. (2002). *Toward a psychology of awakening: Buddhism, psychotherapy, and the path of personal and spiritual transformation*. Shambhala.
14. Chemaly, S. L. (2018). *Rage Becomes Her: the power of women's anger*. Atria Books.
15. Doyle, G. (2020). *Untamed*. Vermilion.
16. Levine, Peter A. (1997). *Waking the Tiger: Healing Trauma: The Innate Capacity to Transform Overwhelming Experiences*. North Atlantic Books.
17. Siegel, Daniel J. (2010). *Mindsight: the new science of personal transformation*. Bantam Books.

PART 3

1. H. Rockcliff, P. Gilbert, K. McEwan, S. Lightman, D. Glover (2008). 'A pilot exploration of heart rate variability and salivary cortisol responses to compassion-focused imagery', in *Clinical Neuropsychiatry*, volume 5, p. 131–139
2. Neff, K. and Christopher K. Germer (2018). *The Mindful Self-Compassion Workbook: A Proven Way to Accept Yourself, Build Inner Strength, and Thrive*. Guildford Press.
3. Germer, C.K. (2009). *The Mindful Path to Self-Compassion: Freeing Yourself From Destructive Thoughts and Emotions*. Guildford Press.
4. Real, T. (2018). *Fierce Intimacy*. Sounds True.
5. Ellen Vora (2022). *The Anatomy of Anxiety*, Orion Spring.
6. Glover Tawwab, N. (2021) *Set Boundaries, Find Peace: A Guide to Reclaiming Yourself*. Hachette.
7. Nagoski, A. and E. (2020). *Burnout: The Secret to Unlocking the Stress Cycle*. Vermilion.
8. Rogers, C. R. (1995). *On Becoming A Person* (2nd ed.). Houghton Mifflin.

ACKNOWLEDGEMENTS

Thank you to Andy, you're my greatest cheerleader and this book wouldn't exist without you. Thank you for taking care of me in big and small ways, and for believing in me before I did. I love you so much.

Thank you to Liv for a lifetime of support, encouragement and belly laughs. Your unwavering faith in me kept me going when things felt heavy. I couldn't do life without you.

Thank you to my agent, Oscar Janson-Smith, for seeing the potential in this book, for truly listening to me, and for supporting me through a few hormonal wobbles! I am very grateful for everything you do.

A giant thank you to the whole Ebury team – in particular Lizzie Dorney and Jessica Cselko, for bringing *Reclaiming You* to life. Thank you to Fearne Cotton for seeing my vision for this book. Thank you to my spectacular editor, Ru Merritt, for the immense passion, care and skill you brought to every chapter of this book. Thank you to Anya Hayes, I'm grateful to have been in such safe and expert hands. Thank you to Anna Morrison for 'getting it' and designing a beautiful cover that I'm immensely proud of. And to Jonathan Baker for the fabulous design and typesetting.

Thank you to all of my clients. You are my greatest teachers and it's a privilege to witness your strength and vulnerability.

Thank you to my community on Instagram for inspiring me to write this book.

I owe immense gratitude to great thinkers like Stephen Porges and Deb Dana. This book simply wouldn't exist without their insights on the nervous system.

Thank you to Christine, for helping me find my voice and reclaim my life.

Thank you to Paul and Doreen for being a source of stability and a model of loving parenting. I learn so much from you and I promise to give your grandchild the same gift you gave your children: unconditional love.

To Julia, thank you for the warmest friendship, the laughs, the 2 a.m hangs, and for walking the hard path with me. I am so grateful.

To Lucy, thank you for your kindness, humour and wisdom, and for 15 years of deep friendship.

To Cat, thank you for making me feel mothered and for helping me believe that I deserve good things.

Thank you to my tutor, Anne Marie Keary – you gave me my first taste of this work. The way you taught body psychotherapy – with such warmth, embodiment and passion – is the reason I pursued this type of therapy.

Thank you to my wonderful supervisor, Athena Matheou, who shaped the therapist I am today. Thank you for your empathy, for countless 'where do you feel it in your body' moments, and for keeping me honest. You are brilliant and your clients and students are so lucky to have you in their lives.

ABOUT THE AUTHOR

Abby Rawlinson is an integrative therapist with a private practice based in east London, UK. Her work mixes traditional psychotherapeutic theories with cutting-edge, evidence-based techniques into a style that feels relatable, down-to-earth, and compassionate. Abby regularly contributes to articles, including but not limited to *Stylist*, *Elle*, BBC, *Harpers Bazaar*, Sheerluxe, *Women's Health*, and *Psychologies*. She can be found on Instagram @therapywithabby or online at therapywithabby.co.uk

NOTES

NOTES